Contemporary Topics in Patient Safety - Volume 2

Edited by Philip N. Salen
and Stanislaw P. Stawicki

Published in London, United Kingdom

Contemporary Topics in Patient Safety - Volume 2
http://dx.doi.org/10.5772/intechopen.104171
Edited by Philip N. Salen and Stanislaw P. Stawicki

Contributors
Deborah Debono, Joanne F. Travaglia, Hamish Robertson, Griselda Gonzalez-Caminal, Aida Camps Gomez, Carmen Gomar-Sancho, Michael Buist, Georgia Arnold, Sunil Jain, Prem Kamal Jain, Arvind Singh Kushwaha, Bhagya Kamal Jain, Abby White, Christopher Kustera, Bryan R. Wilson, Ashley Woodrow, Grace M. Arteaga, Pablo Moreno Franco, Lilia Bacu, Laura Monteiro Viegas, Fátima Moreira Rodrigues, Thomas Nappe, Clayton Korson, Rabbinu Rangga Pribadi, Philip Salen, Stanislaw P. Stawicki

First published in London, United Kingdom, 2023 by IntechOpen
IntechOpen is the global imprint of INTECHOPEN LIMITED, registered in England and Wales, registration number: 11086078, 5 Princes Gate Court, London, SW7 2QJ, United Kingdom

British Library Cataloguing-in-Publication Data
A catalogue record for this book is available from the British Library

Additional hard and PDF copies can be obtained from orders@intechopen.com

Contemporary Topics in Patient Safety - Volume 2
Edited by Philip N. Salen and Stanislaw P. Stawicki
p. cm.
Print ISBN 978-1-83768-134-1
Online ISBN 978-1-83768-135-8
eBook (PDF) ISBN 978-1-83768-136-5

For EU product safety concerns:
IN TECH d.o.o., Prolaz Marije Krucifikse Kozulić 3, 51000 Rijeka, Croatia,
info@intechopen.com or visit our website at intechopen.com.

Meet the editors

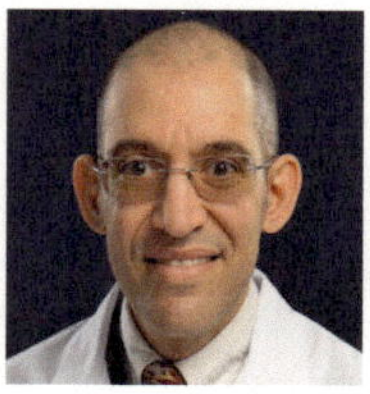

Dr. Philip N. Salen, MD, is an emergency medicine attending and core academic faculty at the St. Luke's University Hospital Emergency Medicine Residency, USA. He is the director of research for the St. Luke's EM Residency and an adjunct clinical associate professor in the Department of Emergency Medicine, Lewis Katz School of Medicine, Temple University, USA. A specialist in emergency medicine, Dr. Salen has co-authored more than 110 scholarly works including journal manuscripts, book chapters, e-book chapters, abstracts, and photo publications. Dr. Salen is a member of multiple editorial and review boards. His areas of expertise include emergency medicine sonography, medical education, patient safety, gastroenteritis, feeding tube complications, radiation safety, and improving emergency medicine clinician communication and wellness.

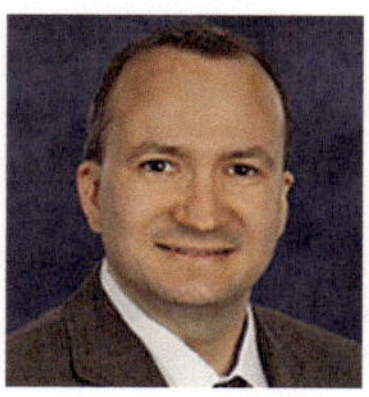

Dr. Stanislaw P. Stawicki, MD, MBA, is a Professor of Surgery and chair of the Department of Research and Innovation, St. Luke's University Health Network, USA. A specialist in trauma, general surgery, and surgical critical care, he has co-authored nearly 700 scholarly works, including more than 25 books. In addition to national and international medical leadership roles, Dr. Stawicki is a member of numerous editorial boards and grant evaluation/review bodies. His areas of expertise include patient safety, medical innovation, blockchain technology, medical education, academic leadership, mentorship, trauma/critical care, and sonography.

Contents

Preface

Patient safety continues to be one of the most important and challenging priorities for healthcare systems around the globe. More than two decades of high-intensity research and administrative, and institutional culture changes have resulted in measurable and significant improvements. Despite this, the attainment of a "zero defect" or "perfect score" patient safety environment remains an elusive target.

As our collective understanding of the importance – and the integral role – of patient safety in everyday clinical practice matures, our ability to ask increasingly more relevant clinical and safety system design questions also grows. Consequently, modern patient safety systems can hardwire process improvement into the very fabric of their day-to-day operations. This, in turn, provides us with continuous opportunities to engage in the journey to "zero defect" and ultra-safe healthcare environments.

Another essential component of the modern patient safety paradigm is the ability to approach complex events associated with often very serious morbidity and even mortality in a fashion that is objective, nonjudgmental, and constructive. The old paradigm of "assigning blame" and "moving on" has given way to the new paradigm of evidence-based, open-minded, and outcome-driven analytical group approaches. Critical thinking, open communication, and the ability of any team member to voice patient safety concerns are all central to our ability to provide clinical care of the highest quality and optimal value.

Without exception, every healthcare provider should strive to attain the mastery of key principles of clinical patient safety, with a focus not only on theoretical considerations but also on practical, everyday bedside implementations of this essential knowledge. Institutional environments continue to evolve toward interactive architectures that facilitate teamwork by way of enhanced communication skills, communal regard among all clinical and non-clinical care providers, and rigorous professionalism. Clinicians and administrators alike must openly encourage and praise behaviors that actively contribute to the establishment and maintenance of a culture of safety across our institutions. Likewise, organizations should encourage and actively support patient safety champions. Ultimately, patient safety will flourish more as a grassroots endeavor rather than as a top-down mandate.

This book is an easily accessible, practical, and problem-focused resource for healthcare practitioners looking to enhance their patient safety knowledge and related clinical and organizational skills. It is our hope that various novel approaches and new perspectives included in this book will stimulate further patient safety discussions, education, and bedside innovation across our clinics and hospitals.

Philip N. Salen, MD
Department of Emergency Medicine,
St. Luke's University Health Network,
Bethlehem, Pennsylvania, USA

Stanislaw P. Stawicki, MD, MBA
Department of Research and Innovation,
St. Luke's University Health Network,
Bethlehem, Pennsylvania, USA

Chapter 1

Introductory Chapter: Patient Safety Remains an Elusive, Fast-Moving Target

Philip N. Salen and Stanislaw P. Stawicki

1. Introduction

Among the most important aspects when creating, developing, and overseeing healthcare facilities and systems are patient and staff safety [1]. The publication of The Institute of Medicine's *To Err is Human* more than 2 decades ago brought much-needed attention to the issue of patient safety in the United States and worldwide by exposing the previously underappreciated impact of medical errors on patient outcomes and illuminating the potential benefits of enhancing safety as an essential core value by US medical practitioners and within US health care institutions [2, 3]. The report endorsed several important agenda items, most notably: errors occur frequently, they have clinical and financial impact, systems-related pitfalls amplify miscues, and preclusion of errors will enhance patient safety [2].

The underappreciation of the patient safety issue can be clearly seen when examining the original report [2]. The Institute of Medicine (now called the National Academy of Medicine) reported that medical errors resulted in between 44,000 and 98,000 potentially avoidable deaths annually in the US alone, which provided additional impetus to a heightened focus on patient safety both in the US and internationally [2, 3]. To give a real-life perspective, the above range of patient safety-event-attributable mortalities is equivalent roughly to an entire population of a small city, and consistently so, year after year.

The Agency for Healthcare Research and Quality (AHRQ) has promoted patient and public safety by encouraging patient safety research during this time in part by focusing on the delineation of error, hospital accreditation, and healthcare directives [2, 4]. Healthcare leadership both institutionally and clinically has focused on patient safety as a metric, utilizing objective scorecards and pay for performance measures [5, 6]. In the context of this chapter, the definition of the phrase "culture of safety" refers to the sum of individual and group ethos, conducts, behaviors, capabilities, and patterns of practice that reflect the adherence to professional and organizational safe practice standards [7].

The primary intent of this textbook, *Contemporary Issues in Patient Safety Volume 2,* is to present a wide-ranging discussion of various, essential patient safety principles and practices to enhance current patterns and to help create patient safety algorithms, systems, and symbioses necessary for the required advancements in clinical outcomes related to patient and staff safety [8].

2. Challenges of evolving healthcare system complexity

Over the last 20 years, significant progress across our healthcare systems has been made when it comes to clinical knowledge, scientific research, and technological advances. Modern technologies have the potential to play an important role in enhancing patient safety via improving hospital algorithms and methodologies for prevention of patient safety adverse events, such as central venous catheter infections, ventilator-associated infections, surgical site infections, and nosocomial urinary tract infections [9, 10]. The medical literature demonstrates that healthcare errors and detrimental events appear to be associated with the ever increasing complexity of medical care as well as poorly optimized workflows [10]. With escalating focus on the centrality of the patient as the core constituent in the clinical safety arena, promoting salubrious practices while eliminating deleterious patterns of expanding healthcare complexity have the potential to facilitate patient safety [8].

Novel implementations of advances in medical knowledge, new medical techniques, and innovative devices empower physicians to provide better, more effective care. However, this sometimes comes at the cost of greater complexity of care. In the process, new contemporaneous challenges may emerge, including the necessity to constantly keep abreast of the latest medical scientific discoveries and devices, further incorporate the ever-expanding role of electronic health records (EHR), and integrate a myriad of new parameters into daily clinical practice, perhaps without fully considering the effects of information overload on the ability to effectively process critical information [11, 12]. Among the unforeseen consequences of this tremendous systemic growth and development is the appearance of situational circumstances that are nearly impossible for a single individual to comprehend, analyze, and act upon. In response to the impact of the rapid increase of complexity of technology on patient safety, many potential solutions have focused on team-based approaches as a foundational value of modern patient-safety approaches [13, 14].

The institutional practice climate has gradually evolved toward a framework that encourages teamwork via emphasis on better communication skills, professionalism, and communal respect among all the clinical and nonclinical care providers [15]. The relationship between patient-safety culture and teamwork has been studied quite extensively in the most complex of hospital environments, critical care units, and other clinical environments to help determine if this relationship improves patient outcomes and impacts staff satisfaction (and safety) [7]. Although differences exist between critical care units in terms of housestaff training versus no housestaff, private versus public, closed versus open "workflow architecture," intensivist versus non-intensivist staffed, and cardiac versus surgical versus neurological versus medical units, team-based approaches within these units have both enhanced perceptions of safety and correlated with beneficial clinical outcomes, staff satisfaction, and staff retention [7, 13].

3. Focus on data quality and high-fidelity event reporting

Among the most crucial issues in patient and staff safety today is the necessity for accurate and non-judgmental reporting (and subsequent discussion) of patient and staff safety events and incidents [6]. While many systems exist for reporting safety incidents, medical errors often go unreported or underreported [16]. A major challenge to accurate reporting of safety miscues is the vulnerability of the so-called "cognitive reality" toward bias and error [17]. Poor or incomplete understating of patient safety issues results in more inaccurate and less relevant epidemiological information available to medical group practices and healthcare organizations, thus hindering key efforts to reduce potential and actual harm to patients [16]. There are multiple barriers to reporting safety incidents, at individual, team, and systemic levels. More specifically, among opportunities to improve safety incident reporting, clinicians note that insufficient feedback to the reporter and anxiety related to reporting occur quite commonly and correspond with low participation rates and less reliable safety data. Notably, physicians are less likely than nurses to document safety incidents [16].

Ex se intellegitur, the accuracy of any reported data will depend heavily on a variety of factors, including the reporting environment and the way any such reporting is handled at the organizational level. The ability to effectively demonstrate and reassure that non-punitive, constructive approaches to addressing patient safety events are hardwired into the organizational fabric is of critical importance. Indeed, this philosophy of dealing with patient adverse event reporting and root cause analysis is known to result in the best overall outcomes and system-wide improvements [15]. Highly structured approaches that incorporate constructive and synergistic learning are required, with recognition of the fact that a vast majority of medical errors have multiple "contributory inputs" and very rarely can be attributed to a single individual and/or action [18]. It is also critical to acknowledge that rigidly hierarchical systems (e.g., top-down command and control environments) will inherently have more potential failure modes than more horizontal systems (e.g., matrix-like partnerships with equally weighted stakeholder inputs) [19].

4. Enhancing safety through role models, teamwork, and leadership

Critical to the successful implementation of such self-learning and self-improving systems is the introduction of patient safety champions or individuals who actively promote patient safety within and across the organizational fabric [8]. These patient safety champions constitute a group of essential role models for other clinicians to emulate and provide sage insight into enhancing patient safety throughout healthcare organizations. The utilization of quality improvement measures directed at promoting the culture of safety and teamwork, for example in decreasing nosocomial hospital acquired infections, has resulted in improved patient care and non-trivial cost reductions [20]. In response to the constantly increasing complexity of healthcare in both inpatient and outpatient arenas, enhancing medical teamwork can improve patient safety and care by offering varying sources of input and knowledge to resolve complex safety issues, make prudent decisions, and complete tasks more productively and efficaciously [21]. Working in concert with patient safety champions, healthcare network's leadership must promote favorable patient safety practices, thereby promoting a well-integrated and comprehensive system of patient safeguards [6]. Properly organized, effective health system leadership necessitates that at every level of medical care delivery (unit, division, department, hospital, and health system), an organizational framework for safety and practice-based improvement exists that interacts effectively and efficiently across the entire matrix of care [11]. Pay-for-performance, a payment model that links quality of care with a corresponding level of payment for healthcare services, reinforces the patient safety role model in that the best performing clinicians will be more fully recognized for better, safer individual (and thus group) outcomes [22] **Figure 1**.

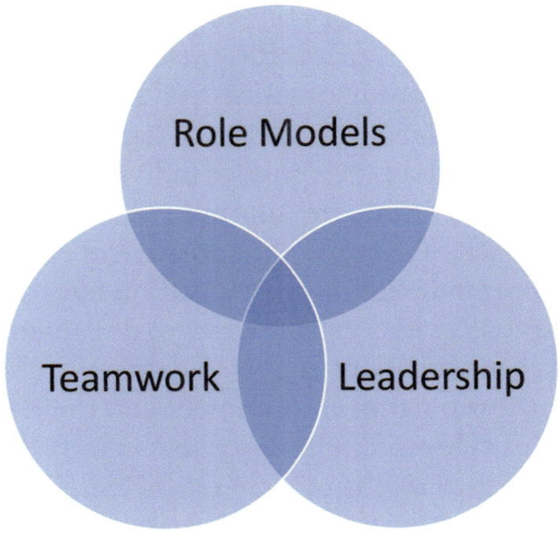

Figure 1.
Improving patient safety via role models, teamwork, and leadership.

5. Enhancing safety via utilization of the electronic medical record, medication ordering algorithms, and artificial intelligence

Health systems with built-in mechanisms for system-wide learning and improvement tend to perform better in general and especially so in the area of patient safety [23]. The Wired for Health Care Quality Act of 2005 appropriated funding in the US to promote adoption of medical information technology to enhance patient safety and improve quality of care [10]. As a consequence, healthcare networks have committed billions of dollars into the adoption of EHR systems, supposing that these systems would transform the incorporation of science-based practices into medical care, thereby resulting in better, safer care at reduced costs [12]. Highly effective and safe healthcare institutions promote and operate safely in multifaceted clinical milieus despite inherently complicated procedures and the potential for error [19]. The implementation of EHR has enhanced communication between providers systemically throughout the healthcare network and between the different specialties while limiting diagnostic errors through utilization of artificial intelligence algorithms [8]. Ongoing plans to maximize medical information technology as a method to incorporate the best science into the clinical arena incorporates decision-making guidance adjuncts, such as specialized disease order sets, documentation guidelines, and best practice algorithms [12].

6. Synthesis and conclusion

The evolution of best performing healthcare systems relies on all the essential elements presented in this textbook, including patient safety education, team-based approaches, accurate safety data collection and processing, the development of patient safety champions, as well as non-judgmental, self-learning, and self-correcting systems. Despite significant improvements during the past two decades, the achievement of sustained zero-defect patient safety performance continues to be as elusive as ever. With increasingly complex healthcare systems, where information and technology tend to evolve faster than an average clinician-stakeholder's ability to "absorb and adjust," our hopes for perfect safety record have become replaced with the realization that the Reason's "Swiss cheese" model applies to complex systems as much as it does to relatively simpler situations and events. Our quest continues toward better, safer healthcare systems. It is a life-long quest that increasingly takes on a form of self-discovering, continually improving organizations, rather than a "once-and-done" achievement of the ever-elusive perfection.

Author details

Philip N. Salen[1*] and Stanislaw P. Stawicki[2]

1 Department of Emergency Medicine, St. Luke's University Health Network, Bethlehem, Pennsylvania, USA

2 Department of Research and Innovation, St. Luke's University Health Network, Bethlehem, Pennsylvania, USA

*Address all correspondence to: philipsalen@gmail.com

References

[1] Green A, Stawicki SP, Firstenberg MS. Introductory chapter: Medical error and associated harm-the critical role of team communication and coordination. In: Firstenberg M, Stawicki SP, editors. Vignettes in Patient Safety. Vol. 3. London, UK: IntechOpen; 2018. pp. 1-14

[2] Bates DW, Singh H. Two decades since to err is human: An assessment of progress and emerging priorities in patient safety. Health Affairs. 2018;**37**(11):1736-1743

[3] Institute of Medicine, Institute of Medicine, Board on Health Care Services, et al. Committe on data standards for patient safety. In: Board on Health Care Services. Patient Safety: Achieving a New Standard for Care. National Academies Press; 2004

[4] Meyer GS, Battles J, Hart JC, Tang N. The US agency for healthcare research and quality's activities in patient safety research. International Journal for Quality in Health Care. 2003;**15**(Suppl. 1):i25-i30

[5] McFadden KL, Henagan SC, Gowen CR. The patient safety chain: Transformational leadership's effect on patient safety culture, initiatives, and outcomes. Journal of Operations Management. 2009;**27**(5):390-404

[6] Green A, Stawicki SP, Firstenberg MS. Introductory chapter: Medical error and associated harm vignettes in patient safety. In: Firstenberg MS, Stawicki SP, editors. Vignettes in Patient Safety. Vol. 3. London, UK: IntechOpen; 2014. pp. 65-72

[7] Dunstan E, Cook JL, Coyer F. Safety culture in intensive care internationally and in Australia: A narrative review of the literature. Australian Critical Care. 2019;**32**(6):524-539

[8] Tolentino JC, Martins N, Sweeney J, Marchionni C, Valenza P, McGinely TC, et al. Introductory chapter: Developing patient safety champions. In: Stawicki SP, Firstenberg MS, editors. Vignettes in Patient Safety. Vol. 2. London, UK: IntechOpen; 2018. pp. 1-23

[9] Middleton B, Bloomrosen M, Dente MA, et al. Enhancing patient safety and quality of care by improving the usability of electronic health record systems: Recommendations from AMIA. Journal of the American Medical Informatics Association. 2013;**20**(e1):e2-e8

[10] Harrison JP, Daly MA. Leveraging health information technology to improve patient safety. Public Administration and Management. 2009;**14**(1):218-237

[11] Pronovost PJ, Mathews SC, Chute CG, Rosen A. Creating a purpose-driven learning and improving health system: The Johns Hopkins medicine quality and safety experience. Learning Health Systems. 2017;**1**(1):e10018. DOI: 10.1002/lrh2.10018

[12] Genies MC, Biondi EA, Berenholtz SM. Leveraging health information technology in the quest to improve health care value. Quality Management in Health Care. 2019;**28**(1):63-64

[13] Taylor N, Zighelboim I, Sholevar F, Stawicki SP, Firstenberg MS. Introductory chapter: Teams in healthcare-a voyage from 'Nice to have' to "the way to go.". In: Firstenberg M, Stawicki S, editors. Teamwork in Healthcare. London, UK: IntechOpen; 2021

[14] Stawicki SP, Cook CH, Anderson III HL, et al. Natural history of retained surgical items supports the need for team training, early recognition, and prompt retrieval. The American Journal of Surgery. 2014;**208**(1):65-72. DOI: 10.1016/j.amjsurg.2013.09.029

[15] Stawicki SP, Firstenberg MS. Introductory chapter: The decades long quest continues toward better, safer healthcare systems. In: Firstenberg MS, Stawicki SP, eds. Vignettes in Patient Safety. London, UK: IntechOpen; 2017:1-14

[16] Noble DJ, Pronovost PJ. Underreporting of patient safety incidents reduces health care's ability to quantify and accurately measure harm reduction. Journal of Patient Safety. 2010;**6**(4):247-250

[17] Croskerry P. The importance of cognitive errors in diagnosis and strategies to minimize them. Academic Medicine. 2003;**78**(8):775-780

[18] Holmström AR. Learning from Medication Errors in healthcare: How to make medication error reporting systems work? Helsingin yliopisto; 2017. Accessed October 9, 2022. Available from: https://helda.helsinki.fi/handle/10138/179230

[19] Portner M, Fumanti BJ, Bendas C, Cipolla J. Learning from others: Examples from air transportation and industrial realms. In: Stawicki SP, editor. Fundamentals of Patient Safety in Medicine and Surgery. Vol. 1. Wolters Kluwer Health (India) Pvt. Ltd; January1 2015. pp. 89-98

[20] Jain M, Miller L, Belt D, King D, Berwick DM. Decline in ICU adverse events, nosocomial infections and cost through a quality improvement initiative focusing on teamwork and culture change. Quality & Safety in Health Care. 2006;**15**(4):235-239

[21] Mayo AT, Woolley AW. Teamwork in health care: Maximizing collective intelligence via inclusive collaboration and open communication. AMA Journal of Ethics. 2016;**18**(9):933-940

[22] Corrigan K, Ryan RH. New reimbursement models reward clinical excellence: Pay-for-performance means that quality and revenue are no longer separate issues for healthcare providers. Healthcare Financial Management. 2004;**58**:88+

[23] Hollnagel E. Braithwaite J. Resilient Health Care: CRC Press; 2019

Chapter 2

Safety in the Home Care Environment of Families Caring for the Elderly

Laura Monteiro Viegas and Fátima Moreira Rodrigues

Abstract

Background: The family is the main provider of care for the elderly, which generates stress, with negative effects on the caregiver's health. It is necessary to relieve the stress of caregivers for the safety of the caregiver and the dependent family member. *Objective*: To evaluate the effect of a nursing intervention based on a psychoeducational program for caregivers of elderly family members. *Methods*: This is a quasi-experimental study, with a sample of caregivers (n = 77), distributed between the intervention group (n = 37) and the control group (n = 40). The instruments comprised a questionnaire with the Zarit Burden scales and the Carers Management Assessment Index. The intervention group benefited from the psychoeducational program, and the control maintained the usual care. *Results*: The intervention group increased coping and decreased the burden compared to the control group. After six months, both groups decreased coping, but it was lower in the intervention group compared to the control group. The intervention group slightly decreased the burden while the control group increased it. *Conclusions*: The nursing intervention is a procedure that relieves the caregiver's burden and increases the coping, contributing to reduce the impact of the damage caused by the provided care.

Keywords: patient safety, domiciliary care, caregivers, frail elderly, nursing

1. Introduction

In 2021, the global patient safety action plan 2021–2030 [1] was approved at the 74th World Health Assembly [1], continuing the process started in 2002, which anticipates the presentation of a report to monitor the implementation progress of this action plan at the 76th World Health Assembly in 2023 [2]. Patient safety is a framework of organized activities that creates cultures, processes, procedures, behaviors, technologies, and environments in health care that consistently and sustainably lower risks, reduce the occurrence of avoidable harm, make errors less likely, and reduce its impact when it does occur [1].

The topic of patient safety generates debates worldwide, aiming at defining the best practices in healthcare environments [3].

Many families provide care for dependent elderly people in the home environment, where there are many dangers. Providing care at home poses risks to the safety of families, who do not know how to organize themselves to provide safe care. Health professionals should assess the caregiver's knowledge and skills, providing guidance on care to ensure that the patient receives safe, quality care and has access to community resources [4].

Clinical practices based on scientific evidence should be implemented to ensure quality on three fronts: improving the health of the individual patient, improving the quality of health care, and strengthening the overall health system [5].

This study aims to disclose the effect of a nursing intervention based on a psychoeducational program for family caregivers of the elderly aiming at reducing burden and improving coping. Caregivers must learn to be competent to manage their own safety and that of elderly family members.

Due to the increase in life expectancy, the last years of life are usually lived with a loss of physical or mental independence, so older people need help and care to perform the activities of daily living (ADL), with the family being the main caregiver [6]. It is inevitable to burden the family caregiver (FC) who transitions from an apparently healthy person to a sick one [7].

Family caregivers constitute a risk group, as they are more vulnerable to the development of physical and psychological morbidities [8], sleep disturbances, abuse, or abandonment of the person cared for. Caring for the elderly requires caregivers to use more health care resources and has inevitable implications for health systems and employing organizations [9].

Collaborating with the family, caregiver in the health system entails the creation of support networks and monitoring by health teams [10] with structured and contextualized interventions so that they can develop more appropriate coping strategies [11].

The dynamic process of caring over time allows the caregiver to learn how to care and acquire skills to perform tasks, care for, and mobilize resources, according to the evolution of the elderly's comorbidities [12].

The model used in this study was the Neuman systems model [13], which contributed to understanding how variables influence a changing client system (consisting of the family caregiver and the dependent elderly). Nursing can help individuals and families maintain their well-being by providing interventions that reduce stressors and adverse conditions that affect the optimal functioning of the client system. Neuman's systems model evaluates the interaction of five variables (physiological, psychological, sociocultural, spiritual, and developmental) in the constantly changing environment, caused by stress factors associated with care. The five client system variables can be located at different levels of the system from the center or core to the lines of resistance (LR) or lines of defense: Normal line of defense (NLD) and flexible line of defense (FLD) [13].

Stressors can arise in the internal or external environment of the family, which are stimuli or forces that create tension and can affect the client system to a greater or lesser degree, causing instability (**Figure 1**) [13].

The nursing actions aim to improve, retain, achieve, or maintain the client's health or well-being, using the three levels of prevention as interventions to keep the system stable. Community nursing cares for family caregivers of the elderly helps them to play their role, improve coping, learn new skills, and face the challenges of daily care [14].

There is evidence of the positive effects of a psychoeducational approach supported by programs for family caregivers in the home environment [15]. In psychoeducation, caregivers learn adaptive skills to deal with care demands and the stress, using a structured format that is usually taught in small groups, including time

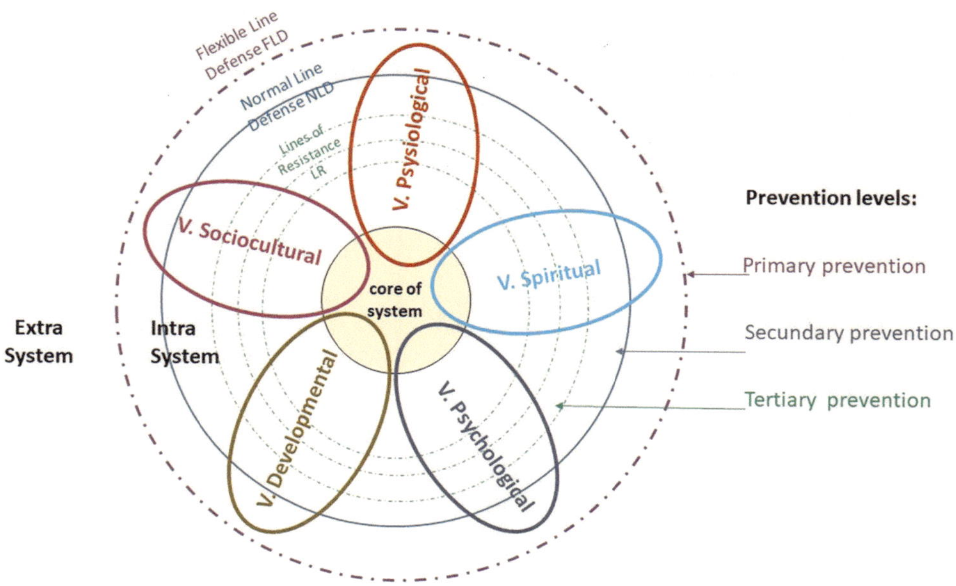

Figure 1.
Neuman's systems Modelan's.

for teaching and practice. The addressed topics typically, include information about dementia, community resources and services, learning to take time to care for oneself, improving communication with family, and skills to manage problem behaviors, such as dealing with negative feelings by managing anger and anxiety, modifying one's way of thinking, and learning to program enjoyable events [16].

This research is a quasi-experimental study, which was carried out based on a pilot study [17] and was based on the following research question: Does the nursing intervention focused on educational and support actions for the family caregiver have an effect on the client system variables (family caregiver and dependent elderly)?

2. Methods

2.1 Sampling and recruitment

The participants are family caregivers of elderly individuals who receive home care from a community health unit. This is an intentional sample and depended on the participants' availability and willingness. The study was carried out from May 2015 to May 2017.

The inclusion criteria comprised adult family members responsible for care and with a score ≤16 on the screening scale for caregivers at risk of burden [18].

To facilitate access to the sample, the researcher joined the nursing team that provides care in the home context and knows the families well. Two groups were organized: the control group (CG), which received the usual care and did not adhere to the program and the intervention group (IG) in which the participants adhered to the intervention based on the psychoeducational stress management program [18]. According to **Figure 1**, after the screening, the sample of 77 participants was organized into two groups, 37 participants from the IG and 40 from the CG, preventing ethical issues since the decision was made by the participants.

The participants underwent a period of continuous assessment for eight months. The 1st evaluation was performed before the intervention (T1 – Baseline), the 2nd evaluation was performed two months after T1 (the intervention in the IG took place during this period) (T2 – post-intervention), and the 3rd evaluation was performed six months after T2 (T3 – follow-up) (**Figure** 2).

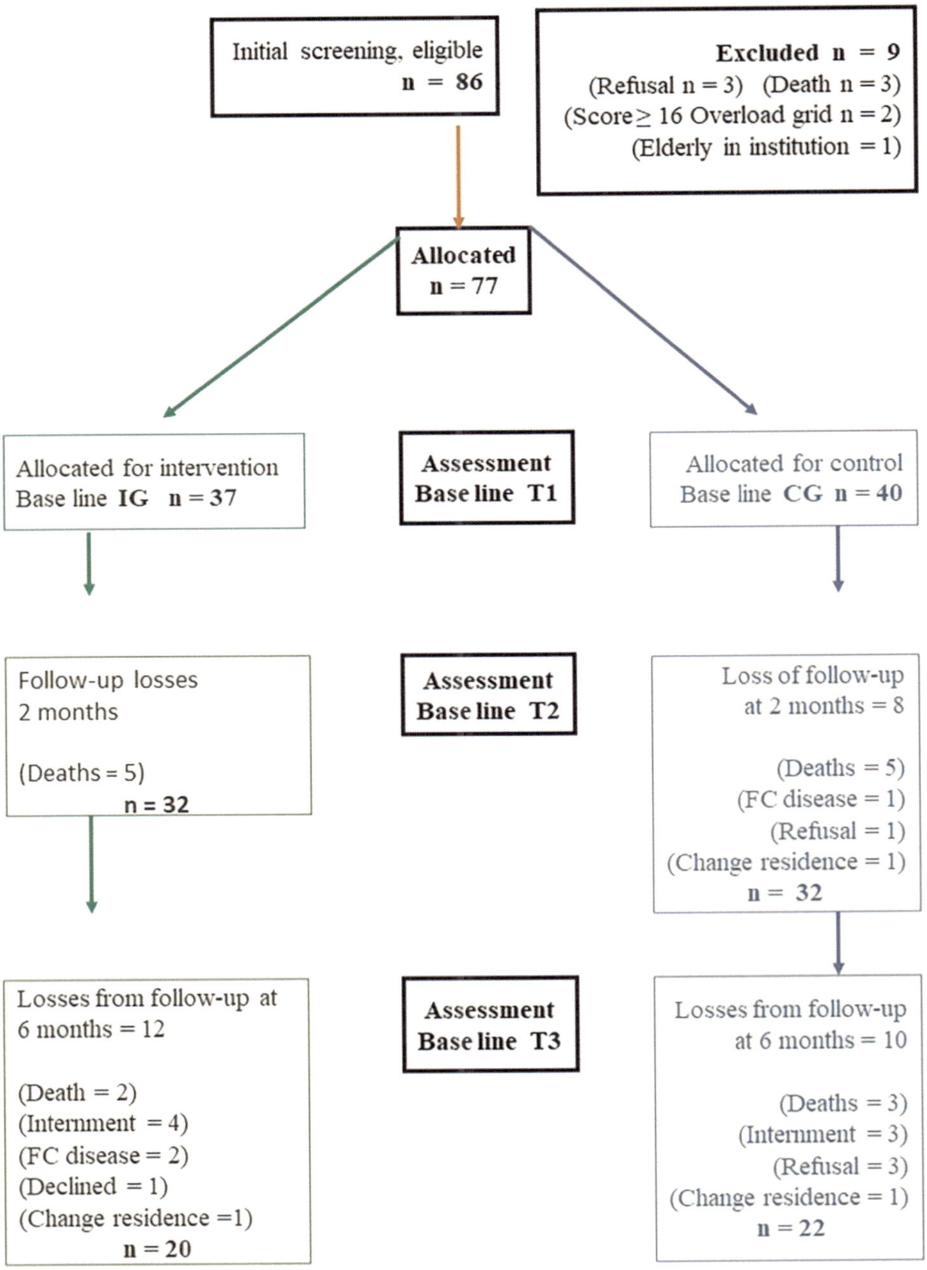

Figure 2.
Participant recruitment and selection flowchart.

The variables of the two client systems were evaluated in three moments: T1, T2, and T3, according to the Neuman System Model, and the comparison between the two groups allowed us to assess the differences in the five variables and at the different levels of the system: core, lines of resistance (LR), and lines of defense (LD). The homogeneity of the results of the characterization variables of the two systems was verified.

2.2 Nursing intervention based on the psychoeducational stress management program.

In the control group (CG), the nurses performed unstructured activities to respond to the difficulties of family caregivers, as usual.

In the intervention group, the nursing team was trained by the researcher to implement the psychoeducational program of the stress management process [18]. They were supported by two documents: "The Caregiver's Guidebook (*Cartilha do Cuidador*) and the "Nurse's Manual" (*Manual do Enfermeiro*).

The stress management program for family caregivers at home aims to help caregivers to develop skills to manage difficult or stressful situations they experience in caring for the elderly at home. The program comprises five steps:

Step 1: Participants' sensitization.

Step 2: Selection of a stressful situation and a goal to be achieved.

Step 3: Situation analysis: This analysis determines the choice of an adapted strategy to be put into practice in the next step.

Step 4: Selection of a strategy adapted to the situation and chosen action, following the presentation of several strategies that can help in the care setting.

Step 5: Evaluation: The final step allows a return to the second step to evaluate how the goal established in that step was achieved. If the goal is not achieved, the stress management process is resumed to allow the caregiver to try another action, which will be evaluated again to direct their thinking until the chosen goal is achieved.

2.3 Hypotheses

Hypothesis 1 – The client system intervention group (IG) shows better results in the variables when compared to the client system control group (CG) at T2 (post-intervention).

Hypothesis 2 – The client system intervention group (IG) shows better results in the variables between moments T2 and T3 when compared to the client system control group (CG).

2.4 Instruments

The data collection instrument was constituted by a questionnaire that includes scales translated and adapted to Portuguese with several parts.

Sociodemographic characterization of the family caregiver and the elderly regarding the following variables: sex, age, marital status, professional status, cohabitation, time of care provision, level of dependence on activities of daily living (ADL) [Basic (ADLB) and instrumental (ADLI)], coping with burden, and social support.

The ADL were assessed through questions, translated, and adapted to Portuguese [19], based on the original questionnaire.

The risk of caregiver burden was assessed by the Carers' Risk Assessment Scale [18]. Caregiver burden was assessed using the Zarit Burden Interview Scale (ZBI). The burden scale values were: no burden (<46), light (47–55), and heavy (>56) [20].

The Caregiver's Coping was assessed by the Carers' Assessment of Management Index (CAMI) [21], translated and adapted to Portuguese [15].

2.5 Statistical analysis

The intervention and the control groups of the client system were compared, using a multiple set of variables, at the three study moments. Initially, descriptive statistics were used: mean, median, standard deviation, coefficient of variation (for quantitative variables, and count of columns and percentages (for qualitative variables), followed by inferential statistics, such as the chi-square test (for qualitative variables) and the comparison of the mean values of the "t-test" (for quantitative variables).

When the conditions for applying the chi-square test were not met for the qualitative variables, Fisher's exact test was used.

The Mann–WhitneyU test was used for quantitative variables when there was no normality between the variables in the 2 groups. The nonparametric *t*-test was used if the normality of the variables in the 2 groups was verified, but their variance was not homogeneous (automatic SPSS procedure).

Both the Kolmogorov–Smirnov test and the Shapiro–Wilk test were used to test the normality of variables in the 2 groups. The significance level was set at 10% [22]. The statistical analysis was performed using the statistical package for the social sciences (SPSS), version 22 (SPSS Inc., Chicago, USA).

2.6 Ethical considerations

Authorization was obtained from the authors of the data collection instruments and the authors of the psychoeducational stress management program to apply them to the clients selected for the study.

The research protocol was approved by the clinical director of the grouping of health units, with favorable opinion n. 093/CES/INV/2014.

The participants were informed about the type of study and after clarification, all of them signed the free and informed consent form (ordinance 015/2013) [23]. The ethical principles of the declaration of Helsinki were considered throughout the process.

During the nursing intervention, ethical care was always ensured, while respecting the family caregiver's availability, individualization of care, belief in their potentials and resources, and the avoidance of value judgments.

3. Results

The two groups were analyzed according to the model systems, regarding the physiological, psychological, sociocultural, and developmental variables in the core and the lines: LR and NLD (**Table 1**).

Statistical homogeneity was verified in the two groups at T1, and the differences observed later can be attributed to the effect of the intervention in the group (IG).

Level	Variables	Variable category	Statistical measures	IG n = 32	CG n = 32	Comparison of groups
Core	Physiological variables					
	Family Caregiver (FC)					
	Age		Average	62.97	63.59	Mann Whitney *p* =.930
			Median	66	66	
			Standard deviation	15.64	13.36	
			Minimum Maximum	24–86	31–86	
	Sex	Female	n (%)	25 (78.1%)	23 (71.9%)	*Fisher's test* *p* =.774
		Male	n (%)	7 (21.9%)	9 (28.1%)	
	Marital status	Married	n (%)	21 (65.6%)	18 (56.3%)	Chi-Square = 1.516 df = 3 *p* =.678
		Single	n (%)	7 (21.9%)	7 (21.9%)	
		Widowed	n (%)	2 (6.3%)	2 (6.3%)	
		Divorced/ separated	n (%)	2 (6.3%)	5 (15.6%)	
	Cohabitation	Yes	n (%)	28 (87.5%)	27 (84.4%)	*Fisher's test* *p* =1.000
		No	n (%)	4 (12.5%)	5 (15.6%)	
	Elderly care					
	Age		Average	81.69	80.34	Mann Whitney *p* =.619
			Median	83.5	81.5	
			Standard deviation	8.69	8.96	
			Minimum Maximum	65–100	65–95	
	Sex	Female	n (%)	15 (46.9%)	17 (53.1%)	Fisher's test *p* =.803
		Male	n (%)	17 (53.1%)	15 (46.9%)	
	Marital status	Married	n (%)	18 (56.3%)	14 (43.8%)	Chi-Square = 3.667 df = 3 *p* = .300
		Single	n (%)	5 (15.6%)	3 (9.4%)	
		Widowed	n (%)	7 (21.9%)	14 (43.9%)	
		Divorced / separated	n (%)	2 (6.3%)	1 (3.1%)	
	Psychological variables					
	Degree of kinship	Spouse	n (%)	14 (43.8%)	12 (37%)	*Chi-Square = .627* *df = 2* *p* =.731
		Son / daughter	n (%)	15 (46.9%)	18 (56.3%)	
		Other	n (%)	3 (9.4%)	2 (6.3%)	
	Sociocultural variables					
	Family Caregiver (FC)					
	Work situation	Employed	n (%)	7 (21.9%)	9 (28.1%)	Chi-Square = .355 df = 3 p = .949
		Unemployed	n (%)	4 (12.5%)	4 (12.5%)	

Level	Variables	Variable category	Statistical measures	IG n = 32	CG n = 32	Comparison of groups
		Retired	n (%)	20 (62.5%)	18 (56.3%)	
		Other	n (%)	1 (3.1%)	1 (3.1%)	
	Schooling	Can read and write	n (%)	0	2 (6.3%)	Chi-Square = 4.836 df = 4 p = .305
		Elementary	n (%)	9 (28.1%)	12 (37.5%)	
		Middle School	n (%)	7 (21.9%)	3 (9.4%)	
		High school	n (%)	5 (15.6%)	7 (21.9%)	
		Higher education	n (%)	11 (34.4%)	8 (25.0%)	
			Elderly			
	Schooling	Illiterate	n (%)	4 (12.5%)	4 (12.5%)	Chi-Square = 8.673 df = 6 p = .193
		Can read and write	n (%)	2 (6.3%)	3 (9.4%)	
		Elementary	n (%)	14 (43.8%)	15 (46.9%)	
		Midlle School	n (%)	4 (12.5%)	4 (12.5%)	
		High school	n (%)	2 (6.3%)	5 (15.6%)	
		Higher education	n (%)	6 (18.8%)	1 (3.1%)	
			Developmental variables			
			Elderly			
		Dependence in activities of daily living (ADL)				
	ADLB		Average	3.1	2.8	Mann Whitney p = .178
			Median	3.4	2.8	
			Standard deviation	0.9	0.9	
			Minimum Maximum	1–4	1–4	
	ADLI		Average	3.5	3.2	Mann Whitney p = .347
			Median	3.9	3.4	
			Standard deviation	0.7	0.7	
			Minimum Maximum	1–4	1–4	
	ADL (total)		Average	46	41.9	Mann Whitney p = .203

Level	Variables	Variable category	Statistical measures	IG n = 32	CG n = 32	Comparison of groups
Normal line of defense (NLD)	Physiological variables					
	Family Caregiver (FC)					
	Degree of risk of burden		Average	11.3	11.6	Mann Whitney p = .542
			Median	11.5	12	
			Standard deviation	2.2	2.1	
			Minimum – Maximum	8–15	8–15	
	How long has the elderly been cared (in years)	Less than 6 months	n (%)	8 (25.0%)	*Chi-Square p* =.877	Chi-Square = 1.792 df = 5 p = .877
		6 months to 1 year	n (%)	3 (9.4%)	5 (15.6%)	
		Between 1 and 3 years	n (%)	9 (28.1%)	8 (25.0%)	
		Between 3 and 5 years	n (%)	2 (6.3%)	4 (12.5%)	
		Between 5 and 10 years	n (%)	5 (15.6%)	3 (9.4%)	
		More than 10 years	n (%)	5 (15.6%)	5 (15.6%)	

Table 1.
Participants' characterization at baseline (T1).

4. Evaluation of the systems in the three evaluation moments

Dependence of the elderly during activities of daily living (ADL).

In the core, the Mann–Whitney test shows a significant difference (p = 0.089) between the IG and CG regarding the ADL at T3. The difference in medians increased at T3 to 0.8, with the CG showing a significantly lower value than the IG. There is a difference in the total ADL, with a relevant variation in the medians at T3: the median in the IG increases from 47 at T2 to 53 at T3, and the CG median decreases from 43 to 24; it was verified that the level of dependence in the CG decreased from very dependent to little dependent.

4.1 Social support

In the LR, the support hours received by the participants increased with time in the IG and decreased in the CG, but there are no statistically significant differences. The IG shows a positive progression of the medians: from 6.5 to 7, between T1 and T3; the CG shows a negative progression of the medians: from 6 to 5, between T1 and T3.

The chi-square test shows statistically significant differences (p = 0.077) between the IG and CG at T3 regarding "who receives support," with the IG receiving more home support. The percentage of support received by caregivers is higher in the IG at the different moments of T1, T2, and T3.

Over time, support hours received by the participants increased in the IG and decreased in the CG. The support provided by the home support center increased for the IG and decreased for the CG. The activity that needs the most support is hygiene care, which increased for the IG and remained the same for the CG throughout the study.

The percentage of caregivers who pay for the support received is lower in all cases in the CG and decreased at T3 in both groups.

4.2 Daily time dedicated to care

Statistically significant differences (P = 0.071) were observed in the NLD with the chi-square test, in the physiological variable at time T2, in the number of hours of care per day, with the IG showing differences when compared to the CG regarding the caregivers who provide care for more than five hours a day.

4.3 Burden

At T1, statistically significant differences in the tests applied to total burden. At T1, the IG and CG groups showed the greatest difference in the median (59 and 51 respectively), with statistically significant differences. The initial differences decrease at T2 and T3, subsequently converging. While the IG decreased the burden between T1 and T2 and maintained the value at T3, the CG results remained the same between T1–T2 and increased at T3. The intervention group had more evident differences, but these differences decreased over the course of the study.

At T1, there were statistically significant differences in the "Expectations of care" category, whose initial values were higher in the IG, and the burden was higher in the IG. However, this initial difference decreased over time (T2 and T3). Nevertheless, it should be noted that over time (T1–T3) they decreased in the IG, while they increased over the same period in the CG. Perceived self-efficacy remained the same at T2 in the IG and decreased in the CG. Over time, it decreased more in the CG than in the IG.

4.4 Coping

Table 2 shows an increase in the coping value (CAMI scale) in the IG when compared to the CG (differences of 5.4 and 4.2 respectively) between moments T1 and T2, meaning that there was an increase in coping after the intervention. At T3, the differences were statistically significant between the two groups after a decrease in the 2 groups. However, this decrease was more prominent in the CG (differences of 14.1 between T2 and T3 in the CG and 6.5 in the IG).

The results show that the intervention group (IG) increased coping and decreased burden compared to the control group (CG). After six months, both groups had decreased coping, but its reduction was lower in the intervention group compared to the control group, with statistically significant differences. The intervention group slightly decreased the burden, while the control group increased it.

NLD Sociocultural Variable	Statistical measures	T1			T2			T3		
		IG	CG	Statistical test	IG	CG	Statistical test	IG	CG	Statistical Test
Coping problem solving	Average	3	3	Mann Whitney p = .707	3.1	3.1	Mann Whitney p = .124	3	2.7	Mann Whitney p = .104
	Median	3	3		3.2	2.9		3.3	2.8	
	S. deviation	0.5	0.4		0.5	1		0.7	0.6	
	Min-Max	2–4	2–4		2–4	2–8		1–4	1–4	
Coping - alternate perception of situation	Average	2.9	2.9	Mann Whitney p = .925	3	3	Mann Whitney p = .506	2.8	2.7	t = .647 p = .522
	Median	2.9	2.8		2.9	1.1		2.9	2.7	
	S. deviation	0.4	0.5		0.6	2.8		0.5	0.6	
	Min-Max	2–4	2–4		2–4	2–8		2–3	1–4	
Coping - dealing with stress symptoms	Average	2.1	2	t = .724 p = .472	2.3	2.3	Mann Whitney p = .199	2.1	1.9	t = .918 p = .364
	Median	2.1	1.9		2.4	2		2	1.7	
	S. deviation	0.6	0.5		0.7	1.3		0.5	0.7	
	Min-Max	1–3	1–3		1–4	1–8		1–3	1–4	
Coping (full scale)	Average	103.3	102.8	Mann Whitney p = .773	108.7	107	Mann Whitney p = .105	102.2	92.9	Mann Whitney p = .099
	Median	105	103		111.5	103.5		106.5	95.5	
	S. deviation	15.3	13.7		16.7	43.6		16.3	28.2	
	Min–Max	63–137	73–123		63–141	0–304		70–125	3–140	

Table 2.
Differences in the two client systems at the three evaluation moments (CAMI scale).

5. Discussion

The profile of family caregivers was defined in both groups, with the mode being female (72% and 78%). The mean age is close to 63 years, a result similar to other studies [7, 24–26]. Most are married women and daughters who live with their parents, as other studies have shown [7, 27–29].

The mean age of caregivers justifies the higher frequency of retired participants. Most are female, which explains the traditional role of women in the family in western society that is associated with caregiver roles. Caregiver daughters are predominant [26]. The fact of being "married" is in accordance with the characteristics of the Portuguese population [30].

In both groups, the elderly have a mean age of 80.3 years, which corresponds to advanced age. Elderly widows in the CG are twice the number found in the IG, which is explained by the predominance of elderly women in the control group, as the average life expectancy of women is higher than that of men [31].

The elderly caregiver in the IG is more dependent regarding the activities of daily living when compared to the elderly in the CG. In both groups, dependence is at the "highly dependent" level, which means that the caregiver takes responsibility for care to support the ADL [24].

There is a similar level of burden risk between the two client systems, with a predominance of moderate risk [31].

In terms of duration of care, most have been caregivers for one to three years. This value is lower than that found in other studies, in which the care duration was more than five years.

Regarding the "daily hours dedicated to care" in the two client systems, the most frequent category is "more than 10 hours a day," which is identical to what was found in other studies [24, 26].

In the present study, at the same evaluation period (T1) we found statistically significant differences in both groups, specifically in the normal line of defense variables of "total burden" (physiological variable) and "caring expectations" (sociocultural variable). The results obtained for these variables in the intervention group show its disadvantage when compared to the control group, but the data also reveal that the elderly were older in the intervention group and were more dependent regarding the activities of daily living.

During the follow-up (T3) the IG client system showed a better assessment of the "global burden", which varied from intense to moderate, while the burden remained moderate in the CG, considering that this change results from the intervention [31].

Also during the follow-up (T3) the study showed the effect of the nursing intervention on coping strategies with statistically significant differences in the IG client system. The intervention facilitated the process that allowed caregivers to find coping strategies with the available resources, focusing on the most effective ones to meet their needs. The intervention allowed the caregivers in the intervention group to focus on the sources from which they received support, when compared to the CG client system. The results show that in the period after the intervention, the intervention group used coping strategies related to the search for support [31].

The greater dependence regarding the ADL in the IG explains the increase in the time spent by the caregiver, when compared to the CG. These differences are statistically significant. The results confirm that the increased ADL dependence by the elderly increases the time of care provision [32].

Due to psychoeducational interventions, caregivers in the intervention group were more empowered, improved social skills, sought support, and disclosed more knowledge of the available resources, which reduces feelings of isolation and stigma [33].

Informal support provided to caregivers declines over time. Nursing guidance is needed to mobilize the community resources and help the system to prevent disruptions and maintain homeostasis [13].

The economic costs of dependent elderly people have increased and the families need help. In the LR at the post-intervention moment (T2), the IG client system increased the percentages of "received support," "payment for received support," "hours of received support," and "home support" in relation to the CG. The increase in these categories occurred over the eight months of the research and is related to the increase in the dependence of the elderly, which has costs associated with care [32].

It is necessary to have policies to support family caregivers. Law N. 100/2019 approves the informal caregiver statute, which regulates the rights and duties of caregivers in Portugal [34].

The health system understands that the family caregiver is a resource, but it is necessary to change the paradigm and understand this is a vulnerable group who needs to be taken care of. The literature refers to the tendency of health professionals to abandon care for less empowered families [34].

At T3, the IG showed the best coping when compared to the CG, with statistically significant differences, which is verified in other studies in which the psychoeducational program was applied [31]. The caregivers must be taught to associate a stressful situation with a coping strategy, making them more effective in the management of difficulties [27].

6. Conclusion

For the caregiver, the responsibility of caring for a dependent elderly family member at home is a stressful situation in the internal and external environment of the client system. Playing the role of caregiver can affect the client system to a greater or lesser degree [17], requiring a different type of intervention by health professionals than is currently provided.

The nursing intervention based on the psychoeducational program is easy, well-structured, and proposes steps to help the caregiver to develop coping strategies that are appropriate to deal with stress factors, promotes the learning of new skills to face the challenges of the care process, helps build confidence to play the role of caregiver, and promotes stability of the client system on the path to well-being.

The present study suggests the advantage of adopting the training program for family caregivers, aiming to minimize the impact of the damage caused by the provided care.

The implementation of the intervention is in line with the strategic objectives of the Global Action Plan on Patient Safety 2021–2030: in objective 1, which aims to reduce avoidable harm to patients to zero; and objective 4, which aims to involve and empower patients and families to help and support them on a safer health care path and contribute to achieve health and well-being goals [3]. The situation experienced at the micro level in the home environment of each family requires health policies and resources organized at the macro level, to reduce the harmful effects for families with dependent members and members who have assumed the role of caregivers.

Conflicts of interest

The authors declare no conflicts of interest.

Author details

Laura Monteiro Viegas* and Fátima Moreira Rodrigues
Department of Community Health at the Lisbon School of Nursing, Portugal

*Address all correspondence to: laura.monteiro@tecnico.ulisboa.pt

References

[1] World Health Organization. Global patient safety action plan 2021–2030: towards eliminating avoidable harm in health care. Geneva: World Health Organization. 2021. Licence: CC BY-NC-SA 3.0 IGO

[2] Order n° 9390/2021 de 24 de setembro de 2021. Aprova o Plano Nacional para a Segurança dos Doentes 2021–2026. Diário da República II Série, N°187(24-09-2021). 96–103

[3] Matos E, Brenda R, Ribeiro R, Sousa B. Teaching patient safety in undergraduate nursing in The State of Bahia. 2021

[4] Given B. Safety of care by caregivers of cancer patients. Seminars in Oncology Nursing. 2019;**35**(4):374-379

[5] Ham-Baloyi WT, Minnie K, Walt VDC. Improving healthcare: A guide to roll-out best practices. African Health Sciences. 2020;**20**(3):1487-1495

[6] Teixeira AR, Alves B, Augusto B, Fonseca C, Nogueira JA, Almeida MJ, et al. Medidas de intervenção junto dos cuidadores informais-documento enquadrador, perspetiva nacional e internacional. Ministério do trabalho e da Segurança Social: Lisbon; 2017

[7] Machado PAP. Papel do prestador de cuidados: contributo para promover competências na assistência do cliente idoso com compromisso do autocuidado. Lisboa: Instituto de Ciências da Saúde da Universidade Católica Portuguesa; 2013

[8] Alzheimer's Association. Alzheimer's disease facts and figures. Alzheimer's Dementia. 2019;**15**(3):321-387

[9] Hopps M, Iadeluca L, McDonald M, Makinson GT. The burden of family caregiving in the United States: Work productivity, health care resource utilization, and mental health among employed adults. Journal of Multidisciplinary Healthcare. 2017;**10**: 437-444

[10] Souza HP, Rodrigues PF, Alcantara RS, Carvalho RA, JHB S, Machado MMP. Physical and emotional impacts on the health care of informal caregivers of patients with Alzheimer's disease. Research, Society and Development. 2021;**10**:16990

[11] Melo R, Rua M, Santos C, Novais S, Mota L, Príncipe F, et al. Intervenção de enfermagem e coping na transição para cuidador familiar. Revista de Investigação & Inovação em Saúde. 2021;**4**(1):61-73

[12] Family Caregiver Alliance. Caregiver assessment: Principles, guidelines, and strategies for change: Report from a National Concensus Development Conference (Vol I). San Francisco: National Center on Caregiving at Family Caregiver Alliance; 2006

[13] Neuman B, Fawcett J. The Neuman Systems Model. 5th ed. New York: Pearson; 2011

[14] Iwasaki T, Yamamoto-Mitani N, Sato K, Yumoto Y, Noguchi-Watanabe M, Ogata Y. A purposeful yet nonimposing approach: How japanese home care nurses establish relationships with older clientes and their families. Journal of family Nursing. 2017;**23**(4): 534-561

[15] Bademli K, Duman Z. Conceptual Framework for nurses in the use the Neuman systems model on caregivers of people suffering by schizophrenia.

International Archives of Nursing and Health Care. 2017;**3**(79):1-5

[16] Cheng ST, Alma A, Losada A, Thompson LW, Gallagher-Thompson D. Psychological interventions for dementia caregivers: What we have achieved, what we have learned. Current Psychiatry Reports. 2019;**21**(7):1-2

[17] Viegas L, Fernandes A, Veiga M. Nursing intervention for stress management in family caregivers of dependent older adults: A pilot study. Revista Baiana Enfermagem. 2018;**32**: e25144

[18] Ducharme F, Trudeau D, Ward J. Manuel de l'intervenant: Gestion du stress: Programme psychoéducatif de gestion du stress destine aux proches-aidants d'un parent âgé à domicile. Montréal: Université de Montréal; 2008

[19] Figueiredo DMP. Prestação familiar de cuidados a idosos dependentes com e sem demência. (Doctoral dissertation). Aveiro: Universidade Aveiro; 2007

[20] Sequeira C. Adaptation and validation of Zarit Burden Interview Scale. Revista Referência. 2010;**12**(3):9-16

[21] Nolan M, Grant G, Keady J. Assessing the Needs of Family Carers: A Guide for Practitioners. Pavilion: Brighton; 1998

[22] Lavrakas P. Encyclopedia of Survey Research Methods. SAGE Publications; 2008

[23] Directorate-General for Health. Norma 015/2013 de 3 de outubro de 2013 – Consentimento informado, esclarecido e livre dado por escrito. Lisboa: Direção Saúde Geral de Saúde; 2013

[24] Custódio JRA. A Sobrecarga e estratégias de coping do cuidador informal do idoso dependente. Coimbra: Instituto Superior Miguel Torga; 2011

[25] Pereira SRD. Cuidar de idosos dependentes. A sobrecarga de cuidadores familiares. Lisboa: Universidade Católica Portuguesa; 2015

[26] Martins J, Barbosa M, Fonseca C. Sobrecarga dos cuidadores informais de idosos dependentes: Caraterísticas relativas ao cuidador. Revista INFAD de Psicologia. 2014;**2**(1):235-242

[27] Ducharme F, Dubé V, Lévesque L, Saulnier D, Giroux F. An online stress management training program as a supportive nursing intervention for family caregiver of an elderly person. Canadian Journal of Nursing Informatics. 2011;**2011**:6

[28] Figueiredo D, Lima MP, Sousa L. Cuidadores familiares de idosos dependentes com e sem demência: rede social pessoal e satisfação com a vida. Psicologia, Saúde & Doenças. 2012;**13**(1): 117-129

[29] Ferreira FEO. A sobrecarga dos cuidadores informais dos doentes de um serviço de oncologia e medicina. (Master dissertation). Lisbon: Instituto de Ciências da Saúde da Universidade Católica Portuguesa; 2012

[30] National Institute of Statistics. Demographic Statistics 2016. Lisboa: National Institute of Statistics; 2017

[31] Ducharme F, Lebel P, Lachance L, Trudeau D. Implementation, and effects of an individual stress management intervention for family caregivers of an elderly relative living at home: A mixed research design. Research in Nursing & Health. 2006;**29**:427-441

[32] Pan X, Lee Y, Dye C, Theriot L. Financial care for older adults with

dementia: Characteristics of adult children's caregivers. The International Journal of Aging and Human Development. 2017;**85**(1):108-122

[33] Cabote CJ, Bramble M, McCann D. Family caregivers' experiences of caring for a relative with younger onset dementia: A qualitative systematic review. Journal of Family Nursing. 2015; **21**(3):443-468

[34] Pereira ICBF. Regresso a casa: Estrutura da acção de enfermagem. Lisbon: Universidade Católica Editora; 2013

Chapter 3

Patient Safety and People Who Are Incarcerated

Hamish Robertson, Deborah Debono and Joanne F. Travaglia

Abstract

We explore a number of key relationships between patient safety and the health status of imprisoned people. This is a conceptual study drawing connections between a number of literatures including the field of patient safety, the work done on health and illness amongst imprisoned people, their social characteristics, and the carceral environment itself. We show that this is an underexplored and under-theorised field of inquiry. It also sets the scene for further investigation of not only individual and systemic factors in the health and illness experienced by such people but the role of the carceral environment. It seems clear that the risk of ill-health rises for many people who are incarcerated. Errors of both omission and commission are common in carceral environments. Risks rise for patients in such environments due to delays in diagnosis, referral and treatment. Understanding the complex and inter-related factors that increase ill-health in individuals, groups and communities provides a starting point for understanding why, when and how imprisoned people need to access and utilise healthcare, how will they are when they do so, and how. It also opens up the question of how these factors might affect their susceptibility to medical errors and adverse events.

Keywords: iatrogenesis, patient safety, carcerality, prisoners, incarceration, social determinants of health

1. Introduction

An exploration of patient safety in this chapter is based on the premise that, just as they contribute to the health status of individuals and populations, social determinants of health contribute to the quality, safety and outcomes of health care. In this chapter we will explore patient safety in this context by exploring the dynamics of the intersection between the carceral environment and the social determinants of health experienced by people who become incarcerated, who are disproportionately from socially marginalised populations vulnerable to poor health outcomes. This chapter examines the intersection between carcerality and patient safety through the complex and inter-related factors that can affect susceptibility to medical error and associated harm(s) for those who are imprisoned. There are broader implications of this work for patient safety in other carceral spaces and places including institutions such as acute psychiatric units and 'locked' dementia wards and for people 'incarcerated' by public health orders.

2. Methodology

This chapter is offered as a conceptual discussion of the issues affecting the quality and safety of care, rather than either an empirical study or a systematic review. The material draws on our research into the quality and safety of care for vulnerable individuals and groups [1] as well as a consideration of the literature we have considered over time. Readers interested in exploring this literature may consider using a range of patient safety terms, such as patient safety, medical or medication error, iatrogenic harm, adverse event, preventable injury, healthcare/hospital acquired infection, nosocomial infection, and or medical harm, as well as terms for incarceration, including for example: prison, incarceration, correctional, jail or gaol, inmate, detention and or parole.

Table 1 provides definitions of some of the key terms relating to incarceration that have been used in this chapter. It must be noted that these terms (their use and definition, including in the specific legal context) may differ from country to country.

3. The health of incarcerated persons

Even prior to their incarceration, people who are incarcerated tend to have worse health than the general population. This can be explained through the lens of the social determinants of health (SDoH), which the World Health Organization explains as the '*the conditions in which people are born, grow, live, work, and age, including the health system. These circumstances are shaped by the distribution of money, power, and resources at global, national, and local levels, which are themselves influenced by policy choices. The social determinants of health are mostly responsible for health inequities—the unfair and avoidable differences in health status seen within and between countries*' [6: n.p.].

Term	Definition
Detention	*Detaining or holding a person charged with a crime following the person's arrest on that charge* [2:61] or *the confinement of a person in custody* [3:199]. Please note that while the first definition appears in the legal and criminology literature, individuals who have not been charged with a crime are also detained by governments, including for example asylum seekers, and people involuntarily admitted to psychiatric hospitals.
Incarceration/carcerality	*Imprisonment in a jail, prison or any penal institution for a period of time ranging from one day to a life-term imprisonment* [2:103].
Jail or gaol or prison	*Prisons are places that house individuals who have been sentenced for violating the criminal law. In some jurisdictions, remand or pre-trial detainees are also incarcerated in prison. Elsewhere, pre-trial detainees are held in jail as opposed to prison. The vast majority of inmates are eventually released from prison; however, prisons provide few rehabilitative opportunities, making re-entry into the wider community very difficult*. [4:171]. There is no consistent agreement in the use of jail/gaol or prison, although jails seem to be associated with shorter term incarcerations, whereas prisons are more often associated with longer term incarcerations.
Parole	*Selective early release from prison followed by supervision.* [5:154]

Table 1.
Terms relating to incarceration.

People who are incarcerated are more likely to have low-income status [7], to be homeless, unemployed, had poor quality education and have poorer health [8, 9]. They are also more likely to be First Nations peoples and/or people with a disability, both groups with worse health than the general population – quite apart from their potential incarceration [9–13] – but these factors act as multipliers of disadvantage [14].

Incarcerated peoples and detainees also have "*... higher rates of mental health conditions, chronic physical disease, communicable disease, tobacco smoking, high-risk alcohol consumption, illicit drug use, and injecting drug use than the general population ... This means that people in prison often have complex, long-term health needs.* [This means that] *the health of people in prison is much poorer compared with the general community, and people in prison are often considered to be elderly at the age of 50–55 (compared with 65 and over in the general community). This is known as 'accelerated ageing'*" [8: 4]. It is important to note that while this quotation is from an Australian publication, the detainees and incarcerated people demonstrate similar patterns of ill health around the globe [14–19], although it should also be noted that knowledge about the health of prisoners demonstrates "*... critical evidence gaps, notably the lack of evidence from low- and middle-income countries*" and in relation to the health of detained adolescents [4, 20].

It is also important to note that while for some incarcerated individuals, prison offers access to healthcare services that were not available prior to incarceration [see for example 21] for most people, incarceration is associated with a worsening of both their mental and physical health [22, 23], including significantly higher "*Rates of infectious diseases, such as tuberculosis, HIV, hepatitis B and C, and sexually transmitted diseases, are higher among the incarcerated population than among the general ... population*" [14: 4S]. This has also been highlighted during the COVID epidemic where factors such as close proximity and delayed or limited prevention strategies [24] mean that "*Carceral facilities are epicenters of the COVID-19 pandemic*" [25: 1].

3.1 Mental health and patient safety of incarcerated person

The mental health of incarcerated individuals is of particular concern, both prior and subsequent to incarceration. The compounding nature of ill-health and incarceration is particularly evident in relation to mental health. As David Satcher argues "*Far too many people enter our criminal justice system due to an untreated or under-treated mental illness. Too often, we find our prison system substituting for the mental health care once provided in mental hospitals and other medical settings. It is estimated that one in six people in the correctional system lives with a serious mental illness. Compounding the problem is the co-occurrence of mental illness and substance abuse*" [26: vi]. Rekrut-Lapa & Lapa [15: 69] speak to a similar conclusion, but also noted that such conditions "*... require both emergency and routine care.*" They also found evidence that about a third of medications possessed by detainees at arrest were for the management of psychiatric illnesses.

Even for people without a prior mental illness, the experience of incarceration can act to facilitate these conditions. One high profile example of this is the rapid mental deterioration of many asylum seekers incarcerated while they await a review of their situation, in detention centres around the world [27, 28]. Commonly reported mental health issues experienced by long term detainees included "*Depression and demoralisation, concentration and memory disturbances, and persistent anxiety ... Standardised measures found high rates of depression, anxiety, PTSD and low quality of life scores*" [29: 2070].

Suicide is also a recurrent risk for incarcerated persons, accounting for about a half of prison deaths worldwide [30] and is 13 times higher in released prisoners than in the general population [31]. Rekrut-Lapa & Lapa [15: 70] quoted a UK report which showed that 46% of near misses (defined as *any incident which resulted in, or could have resulted in, serious illness or self-harm of a detainee*) in police custody were attempted suicides and self-harming behaviour, in contrast to medical emergencies which only made up 14% of such incidents.

4. Carcerality

There is a growing interdisciplinary literature on studies of the process of incarceration itself, on carceral spaces and places, and their consequences for those incarcerated [32]. Such spaces are increasingly seen to include not only places of formal imprisonment but various institutional spaces that may have 'secure' facilities and associated features [e.g. 33, 34]. These may be both formalised and informal (e.g. informal and formal refugee camps) and cover the control and 'management' of various groups in the population e.g. secure youth facilities, mental health facilities, disability care facilities, orphanages and so on. In other words, there is a growing understanding of the similarities between the types of carceral spaces societies produce and the systemic problems that can occur in them.

One of the issues associated with such spaces is that, historically at least, some have been the sites of abusive practices including, for example, Parramatta Girls Home in New South Wales, Australia where young, often Aboriginal, girls were subject to significant physical, psychological and sexual abuses over many decades [see 35, 36]. These types of institutions and their practices effectively manufacture places of abuse and ill-health. And this is far from unique, as many inquiries into patient safety, child abuse and other domains have shown across various jurisdictions [e.g. 37, 38]

This nexus of institutional, carceral spaces has clearly produced a variety of negative outcomes for many of those incarcerated including both physical and mental health consequences as illustrated throughout this chapter. Such outcomes can be long-term, even lifelong, in their impacts making such sites the producers of ill-health for those detained within them. In the criminological literature these forms of often sustained abuses of the rights of individuals have even been characterised as the consequences of harmful societies [39]. This emphasis suggests that our societies have the capacity to generate systemic institutional harms that, ultimately, must reflect back on that society. In effect, the abuses enacted, and tolerated, in carceral spaces reflect the 'true' values of our societies because they represent enacted values in contrast to espoused values [e.g. 40].

To address these types of societal and systemic drivers of abuse in these sorts of bounded carceral environments, we need to consider the voices of those harmed and not simply the official responses or inevitable list of formal recommendations that often result. In other words, we need to disrupt the conventional discourses that present such spaces/places and the abuses that occur within them as exceptions to some general benevolent rule. As various writers have commented, including feminist theorists, this process of exceptionalising often widespread, even repetitive, systemic abuses, adds an additional harm to those injured in them [see 41]. Their experiential truths are often either minimised or dismissed in systemic responses and thus there is a diminution of the harms perpetrated on people who are often amongst the most vulnerable in our societies.

This approach has an additional benefit for both theory and research because it extends the scope of inquiry beyond the individual carceral site and seeks to identify and unpack patterns of health-related harms and their connection to the environments, or places, within which they occur. We would further suggest that there is an issue of *generativity* to be examined here in that some institutions can acquire such reputations but not all do, or at least not to the same degree. If the pattern is not uniform, then clearly some mix of institutional governance and perhaps individual factors combine to enable carceral environments that produce these types of harmful outcomes. This in turn can assist us in developing a body of theory to examine past, present and potentially future scenarios where such problems have emerged and might yet emerge. Potentially, at least, if such understanding can be used to influence policy, practices and professional values then future harms may be averted.

We can look for and potentially predict the consequential outcomes for human health and wellbeing in carceral environments that have the capacity for, or may have even already produced, harms to vulnerable people in them (we note this may include staff too). And we can seek to understand these factors better by looking for similarities and differences across multiple carceral domains – prisons, youth detention, mental health, aged care and so on. By disrupting the systemic distinctions between these often quite similar environments, we can better theorise why such things emerge in this first place and why they persist. In addition, because some causes are obvious to a degree, we can readily identify the repetition of factors that lead to harms.

The current reporting on deaths at the New York Riker's Island facility illustrates how contemporary these issues are and yet how sustained they can be across time to the serious detriment of those incarcerated within them. Examining such facilities on a case-by-case basis runs the serious risk of making each one seems unique when clearly a variety of overt and covert factors are in play.

5. The safety of incarcerated patients

The provision of healthcare to prisoners is a complex task, because as discussed earlier in this chapter, prisoners are often at the intersection of multiple vulnerabilities and multifaceted mental and physical conditions affecting their health [14], with treatments undertaken in an environment which is often not under either the patients' or clinicians' control [42, 43].

The irony of prison health is that in some cases treatment within prisons may be the best opportunity an individual has to receive the care they require [21]. This is 'balanced,' however, by the difficulties and barriers which impede such care and which include everything from societal attitudes to prisoners, to clinicians' knowledge and experience of specific conditions and treatments [44]. In between these two extremes are the difficulties faced in both providing and receiving care when the patient frequently has multiple co-morbidities, including mental health issues [45].

Patient safety is defined as the "*... avoidance, prevention and amelioration of adverse outcomes or injuries stemming from the process of healthcare*" [46: 31], which in turn are defined as injuries caused "*... by medical management (rather than the underlying disease) and that prolonged the hospitalization, produced a disability at the time of discharge, or both*' [47: 370]. There are two broad categories of errors – that is errors of commission (where something wrong was done) and errors of omission (where the right thing was not done) [48: n.p.] and three categories of adverse events: '*Preventable adverse events: those that occurred due to error or failure to apply an accepted strategy for prevention; Ameliorable adverse events: events that, while not preventable, could have been less harmful if care had been different;* [and] *adverse events due to negligence: those* *that occurred due to care that falls below the standards expected of clinicians in the community'* [49: n.p.].

While the available literature is limited, what is available shows clear patterns of errors of omission and commission for incarcerated people. In terms of errors of commission (where the wrong thing was done) the literature shows that the safety of care for incarcerated people is lessened by factors such as: mis-diagnosis [50–52], medication errors/issues [53, 54] including under-prescribing/ceasing medications before indicated by evidence based practice [55: 506] or over-prescribing particularly in the case of women, as a mechanism for control [56–58] and/or polypharmacy [59].

The list of errors of omission are even longer. Studies show that the quality and safety of care for incarcerated individuals is lessened by: failure to diagnose treatable conditions [60, 61]; failure to treat latent infection [62]; fear/lack of confidence in clinicians inhibiting uptake of treatments [63, 64]; and routine failures to identify and mitigate risk factors (particularly in mental health) [65].

A recurrent theme in the literature on errors of omission in prisons is the effects of delays on patient outcomes, including: delays in testing or diagnosis [62, 66, 67]; delays in treatment [56, 61]; and delayed responses to request for medical appointments issues [54].

Patient safety for incarcerated individuals is also notable for the evidence of two factors associated with the particular experience of incarceration itself. These are prisoners' experience of the negative attitudes of clinical staff [68–71], including failures of privacy and lack of dignity/incivility [53, 54, 72] and the way in which treatment is (or is not) provided including: treatment interruption [73, 74]; lack of continuity of care [75]; and the discontinuation of treatment on release from prison [62, 76–80].

6. Improving the quality and safety of care for prisoners

Health providers and services have a legal and moral obligation to provide safe care to people who are incarcerated. The United Nations Mandela minimum rules for the treatment of prisoners includes specific medical and health care requirements. Under the category of vulnerable groups of people, the United Nations state that governments have the responsibility to *"Ensure that prisoners with physical, mental or other disabilities have full and effective access to prison life on an equitable basis, and are treated in line with their health conditions"* [81: 7]. The section on medical and health services underscores that clinicians'*"... relationship with prisoners is governed by the same ethical and professional standards as those applicable to patients in the community"* including: *"ensuring the same standards of health care that are available in the community and providing access to necessary health-care services to prisoners free of charge without discrimination; evaluating, promoting, protecting and improving the physical and mental health of prisoners, including prisoners with special healthcare needs; adhering to the principles of clinical independence, medical confidentiality, informed consent in the doctor-patient relationship and continuity of treatment and care (including for HIV, tuberculosis, other infectious diseases and drug dependence);* [and] *an absolute prohibition of health-care professionals to engage in torture or other forms of ill-treatment, and an obligation to document and report cases of which they may become aware"* [81: 8].

The literature on the quality and safety of care for incarcerated persons also provides insights into potential ways of improving this care. These fall into three broad categories of improved treatment, improved education and training for both health professionals and prisoners, and improved coordination of care. The literature specifically suggests the need to improve the: diagnosis, screening and triage for those entering correctional facilities [51, 52, 64]; medical assessment and care in police custody [54, 82, 83]; therapeutic relationships between inmates and correctional healthcare staff [73, 84]. It also identifies the need to reduce polypharmacy [57], provide alternative mental health treatment other than medication [56], introduce short-course treatment for latent TB infection [74, 77] and the provision of care consistent with TB treatment guidelines [62], and finally allowing the self-administration of treatment by inmates [72, 84].

Other improvement strategies are based on the education of health professionals and or incarcerated persons. These include the need to improve training for healthcare professionals working in correctional facilities [60], including training to improve knowledge and attitudes among custodial staff [e.g. 64, 68, 69, 71, 73] and, on the other hand, the provision of health literacy education programs for incarcerated persons, especially understanding of the importance of adherence to treatment [e.g. 63, 64, 66, 71, 73]. One organisational strategy which has been suggested by numerous studies is the need to improve the co-ordination and communication between correctional and community-based health services to improve health care and continuity of treatment [e.g. 62, 75, 76, 78–80].

Finally, the John Jay College of Criminal Justice in New York proposed a set of patient safety standards for prisons, entitled "Patient Safety Behind Bars". These address most of the requirement of the Mandela rules, and specifically address: access to and the availability of care (including access to prenatal and postpartum care); establishing a culture of safety within the incarcerating organisations (including active safety leadership and a shift to a systems approach to the safety of care); addressing the needs of health care personnel (including training, addressing staff fatigue and burnout, ensuring adequate staffing and competency); medication management (including the use of computerized medication systems); management of transitions and communication (including ensuring timely access to specialists, tests and consultations); addressing specific conditions (ranging from chronic diseases and the provision of access to care after acute mental health problem); and finally the involvement of patients in their care and treatment (including informed consent, informed refusal, the provision of interpreters, patient notification of results, patient tailored decisions and the choice of advanced directives) [85].

7. Conclusion

In this chapter we bring together some of the core issues affecting the safety of care for incarcerated persons. These issues typically begin far earlier than the person's incarceration, in the social determinants of health which affect their communities, families and themselves disproportionately. On entering incarceration, the risk of ill health increases. The provision of safe, quality health care therefore is not just a question of addressing the existing health conditions of inmates, but also of ensuring that they are not exposed to additional iatrogenic harm, as has been the case during the COVID pandemic.

While the literature is somewhat limited, the studies and frameworks which are available provide a clear direction in terms of improving the existing quality of care for people who are incarcerated. Most importantly they point to the need to understand the unique history, context and health risks faced by incarcerated people, both prior and subsequent to their incarceration. Finally, the growing literature on carcerality itself points to new ways of examining and theorising the health effects, both short and long term, of the incarceration experience. This in turn suggests the opportunity for an expanding cross-disciplinary research and knowledge development base as key concepts and tools are applied to a growing variety of carceral environments.

Author details

Hamish Robertson, Deborah Debono and Joanne F. Travaglia*
Centre for Health Services Management, School of Public Health, University of Technology Sydney, Sydney, NSW, Australia

*Address all correspondence to: joanne.travaglia@uts.edu.au

References

[1] Braithwaite J, Travaglia JF, Nugus P. Giving a Voice to Patient Safety in New South Wales. Sydney: Clinical Excellence Commission; 2007

[2] Mushanga M. Dictionary of Criminology. Kampala, Uganda: LawAfrica Publishing; 2011

[3] Allan S et al. LexisNexis Concise Australian Legal Dictionary. 6th ed. Chatswood: Lexis Nexis Butterworths; 2011

[4] Coomber R, Donnermeyer JF, McElrath K, Scott J. Key concepts in Crime and Society. Los Angeles: Sage; 2014

[5] Walsh D, Poole A. A Dictionary of Criminology. Oxford: Routledge; 2019

[6] World Health Organization. About social determinants of health. Geneva: World Health Organization; 2018

[7] Rabuy B, Kopf D. Prisons of poverty: Uncovering the pre-incarceration incomes of the imprisoned. Prison Policy Initiative. 2015;**9**

[8] Australian Institute of Health and Welfare, The Health of Australia's Prisoners 2018. Canberra: Australian Institute of Health and Welfare; 2019

[9] Bryan K. Adults in the Prison Population. In: Cummings L, editor. Handbook of Pragmatic Language Disorders. Switzerland: Springer; 2021. pp. 691-714

[10] Valeggia CR, Snodgrass JJ. Health of indigenous peoples. Annual Review in Anthropology. 2015;**44**(1):117-135

[11] Gracey M, King M. Indigenous health part 1: Determinants and disease patterns. The Lancet. 2009;**374**(9683):65-75

[12] Trofimovs J, Dowse L, Srasuebkul P, Trollor JN. Using linked administrative data to determine the prevalence of intellectual disability in adult prison in New South Wales, Australia. Journal of Intellectual Disability Research. 2021;**65**(6):589-600

[13] Whittingham L et al. The prevalence and health status of people with developmental disabilities in provincial prisons in Ontario, Canada: A retrospective cohort study. Journal of Applied Research in Intellectual Disabilities. 2020;**33**(6):1368-1379

[14] Bui J, Wendt M, Bakos A. Understanding and Addressing Health Disparities and Health Needs of Justice-Involved Populations Public Health Reports. Introductory Research Support. 2019;**134**(1):35-75

[15] Rekrut-Lapa T, Lapa A. Health needs of detainees in police custody in England and Wales. Literature review. Journal of Forensic and Legal Medicine. 2014;**27**:69-75

[16] Kouyoumdjian F, Schuler A, Matheson FI, Hwang SW. Health status of prisoners in Canada: Narrative review. Canadian Family Physician. 2016;**62**(3):215-222

[17] Wolff H et al. Health problems among detainees in Switzerland: A study using the ICPC-2 classification. BMC Public Health. 2011;**11**(1):1-13

[18] Maccio A et al. Mental disorders in Italian prisoners: Results of the REDiMe study. Psychiatry Research. 2015;**225**(3):522-530

[19] Dumont DM, Allen SA, Brockmann BW, Alexander NE, Rich JD. Incarceration, community health, and racial disparities. Journal of Health Care for the Poor and Underserved. 2013;**24**(1):78-88

[20] Kinner SA, Young JT. Understanding and improving the health of people who experience incarceration: An overview and synthesis. Epidemiologic Reviews. 2018;**40**(1):4-11

[21] Mignon S. Health issues of incarcerated women in the United States. Ciencia & Saude Coletiva. 2016;**21**:2051-2060

[22] Brinkley-Rubinstein L. Incarceration as a catalyst for worsening health. Health & Justice. 2013;**1**(1):1-17

[23] Smith SA, Braithwaite RL. Introduction to public health and incarceration: Social justice matters. Journal of Health Care for the Poor and Underserved. 2016;**27**(2A):1

[24] Cervin C. Justice required: Vaccination in Canadian prisons. Canadian Family Physician. 2021;**67**(3):215-215

[25] Strodel R et al. COVID-19 vaccine prioritization of incarcerated people relative to other vulnerable groups: An analysis of state plans. PLOS ONE. 2021;**16**(6):e0253208. DOI: 10.1371/journal.pone.0253208

[26] Satcher D. Foreward. In: Greifinger R, editor. Public Health behind Bars: From Prisons to Communities. 2nd ed. Switzerland: Springer; 2022. pp. v-vii

[27] Robjant K, Hassan R, Katona C. Mental health implications of detaining asylum seekers: Systematic review. The British Journal of Psychiatry. 2009;**194**(4):306-312

[28] van Eggermont Arwidson C, Holmgren J, Gottberg K, Tinghög P, Eriksson H. Living a frozen life: A qualitative study on asylum seekers' experiences and care practices at accommodation centers in Sweden. Conflict and Health. 2022;**16**(1):1-14

[29] Coffey GJ, Kaplan I, Sampson RC, Tucci MM. The meaning and mental health consequences of long-term immigration detention for people seeking asylum. Social Science & Medicine. 2010;**70**(12):2070-2079

[30] Fazel S, Baillargeon J. The health of prisoners. The Lancet. 2011;**377**(9769):956-965

[31] Jones D, Maynard A. Suicide in recently released prisoners: A systematic review. Mental Health Practice. 2013;**17**(3)

[32] Coulson HL. New directions in carceral studies. Journal of Urban History. 2021;**47**(1):202-208

[33] Danely J. What older prisoners teach us about care and justice in an aging world. Anthropology and Aging. 2022;**43**(1):58-65

[34] Repo V. Carceral riskscapes and working in the spaces of mental health care. Fennia. 2020;**198**(1-2):121-134

[35] Franklin C. Belonging to bad: Ambiguity, parramatta girls and the parramatta girls home. Geographical Research. 2014;**52**(2):157-167

[36] Lloyd J, Steele L. Place, memory, and justice: Critical perspectives on sites of conscience. Space and Culture. 2022;**25**(2):144-160

[37] Corby B, Doig A, Roberts V. Public Inquiries into Residential Abuse of Children. London: Jessica Kingsley Publishers; 2001

[38] Hughes M. Towards the inquiry into aged care and beyond: The promise and challenge of a new era in LGBTI ageing. In: Peel E, Harding R, editors. Ageing and Sexualities. London: Routledge; 2017. pp. 183-204

[39] Pemberton SA. Harmful Societies: Understanding Social Harm. Bristol: Policy Press; 2016

[40] English LM. The impact of an independent inspectorate on penal governance, performance and accountability: Pressure points and conflict "in the pursuit of an ideal of perfection". Critical Perspectives on Accounting. 2013;**24**(7-8):532-549

[41] Thiel D, South N. Criminal ignorance, environmental harms and processes of denial. In: Gross M, McGoey L, editors. Routledge International Handbook of Ignorance Studies. London: Routledge; 2022. pp. 334-344

[42] Pont J, Enggist S, Stöver H, Williams B, Greifinger R, Wolff H. Prison health care governance: Guaranteeing clinical independence. American Journal of Public Health. 2018;**108**(4):472-476

[43] MacDonald R, Parsons A, Venters HD. The triple aims of correctional health: Patient safety, population health, and human rights. Journal of Health Care for the Poor and Underserved. 2013;**24**(3):1226-1234

[44] Werner S, Stawski M. Mental health: Knowledge, attitudes and training of professionals on dual diagnosis of intellectual disability and psychiatric disorder. Journal of Intellectual Disability Research. 2012;**56**(3):291-304. DOI: 10.1111/j.1365-2788.2011.01429.x

[45] Bradley L. The Bradley Report: Lord Bradley's Review of People with Mental Health Problems or Learning Disabilities in the Criminal Justice System. London: Department of Health; 2009

[46] Vincent C. Patient Safety. 2nd ed. Chichester, West Sussex: Wiley-Blackwell; 2010

[47] Brennan TA, Leape LL, Laird NM, et al. Incidence of adverse events and negligence in hospitalized patients. Results of the Harvard Medical Practice Study I. New England Journal of Medicine. 1991;**324**:370-376

[48] Agency for Healthcare Research and Quality, Glossary: Error, Rockville, MD.: Agency for Healthcare Research and Quality 2017. [Online]. Available: https://psnet.ahrq.gov/glossary/e. Accessed on: 20 March 2018

[49] Agency for Healthcare Research and Quality, Patient safety primer: Adverse events, near misses and errors, Rockville, MD.: Agency for Healthcare Research and Quality 2017. [Online]. Available: https://psnet.ahrq.gov/primers/primer/34/adverse-events-near-misses-and-errors?q=adverse+event+and+definition. Accessed on: 20 March 2018

[50] Martin MS, Hynes K, Hatcher S, Colman I. Diagnostic error in correctional mental health. Journal of Correctional Health Care. 2016;**22**(2):109-117

[51] Mitchell P, Shaw J. Factors affecting the recognition of mental health problems among adolescent offenders in custody. Journal of Forensic Psychiatry and Psychology. 2011;**22**(3):381-394

[52] Martin MS, Potter BK, Crocker AG, Wells GA, Grace RM, Colman I. Mental health treatment patterns following screening at intake to prison. Journal of Consulting and Clinical Psychology, Article. 2018;**86**(1):15-23. DOI: 10.1037/ccp0000259

[53] Hatton DC, Kleffel D, Fisher AA. Prisoners' perspectives of health problems and healthcare in a US women's jail. Women & Health. 2006;**44**(1):119-136

[54] Kennedy KM, Green PG, Payne-James JJ. Complaints against health-care professionals providing police custodial and forensic medical/ health-care services and sexual offence examiner services in England, Wales and Northern Ireland. Medicine, Science, and the Law. 2017;**57**(1):12-32

[55] Gjersing LR, Butler T, Caplehorn JRM, Belcher JM, Matthews R. Attitudes and beliefs towards methadone maintenance treatment among Australian prison health staff. Drug and Alcohol Review. 2007;**26**(5):501-508

[56] Hassan L et al. Prevalence and appropriateness of psychotropic medication prescribing in a nationally representative cross-sectional survey of male and female prisoners in England. BMC Psychiatry;**16**(1):346

[57] Hassan L, Senior J, Frisher M, Edge D, Shaw J. A comparison of psychotropic medication prescribing patterns in East of England prisons and the general population. Journal of Psychopharmacology. 2014;**28**(4):357-362. DOI: 10.1177/0269881114523863

[58] Kjelsberg E, Hartvig P. Too much or too little? Prescription drug use in a nationwide prison population. International Journal of Prisoner Health. 2005;**1**(1):75-87. DOI: 10.1080/17449200500156871

[59] Griffiths EV, Willis J, Spark MJ. A systematic review of psychotropic drug prescribing for prisoners. Australian and New Zealand Journal of Psychiatry. 2012;**46**(5):407-421. DOI: 10.1177/0004867411433893

[60] Adane K, Spigt M, Ferede S, Asmelash T, Abebe M, Dinant GJ. Half of pulmonary tuberculosis cases were left undiagnosed in prisons of the Tigray region of Ethiopia: Implications for tuberculosis control. PLoS ONE. 2016;**11**(e0149453):2

[61] Vaughn MS. Penal harm medicine: State Tort remedies for delaying and denying health care to prisoners. Crime, Law and Social Change. 1999;**31**(4):273-302

[62] Reichard AA, Lobato MN, Roberts CA, Bazerman LB, Hammett TM. Assessment of tuberculosis screening and management practices of large jail systems. Public Health Reports. 2003;**118**(6):500

[63] de Juan J et al. Reasons for not initating HCV treatment in prison: A subanalysis of the EPIBAND study. Revista española de sanidad penitenciaria, Article. 2011;**13**:44-51

[64] Morgan RD, Steffen J, Shaw LB, Wilson S. Needs for and barriers to correctional mental health services: Inmate perceptions. Psychiatric Services. 2007;**58**(9):1181-1186

[65] Way BB, Kaufman AR, Knoll JL, Chlebowski SM. Suicidal ideation among inmate-patients in state prison: Prevalence, reluctance to report, and treatment preferences. Behavioral Sciences and the Law. 2013;**31**(2):230-238

[66] Crowley D, Van Hout MC, Lambert JS, Kelly E, Murphy C, Cullen W. Barriers and facilitators to hepatitis C (HCV) screening and treatment - A description of prisoners' perspective. Harm Reduction Journal, Art no. 2018;**15**:62. DOI: 10.1186/ s12954-018-0269-z

[67] Rautanen M, Lauerma H. Imprisonment and diagnostic delay

among male offenders with schizophrenia. Criminal Behaviour and Mental Health. 2011;**21**(4):259-264

[68] Clark KA, White Hughto JM, Pachankis JE. "What's the right thing to do?" Correctional healthcare providers' knowledge, attitudes and experiences caring for transgender inmates. Social Science and Medicine, Article. 2017;**193**:80-89. DOI: 10.1016/j.socscimed.2017.09.052

[69] Cuthbertson L, Kowalewski K, Edge J, Courtney K. Factors that promote and hinder medication adherence from the perspective of inmates in a provincial remand center: A Mixed Methods Study. Journal of Correctional Health Care, Article. 2018;**24**(1):21-34

[70] Aday R, Farney L. Malign neglect: Assessing older women's health care experiences in prison. Journal of Bioethical Inquiry, Article. 2014;**11**(3):359-372. DOI: 10.1007/s11673-014-9561-0

[71] Seyed Alinaghi SA et al. Adherence to antiretroviral therapy and tuberculosis treatment in a prison of Tehran, Iran. Infectious Disorders – Drug Targets. 2016;**16**(3):199-203

[72] Roberson DW, White BL, Fogel CI. Factors influencing adherence to antiretroviral therapy for HIV-infected female inmates. Journal of the Association of Nurses in AIDS Care. 2009;**20**(1):50-61. DOI: 10.1016/j.jana.2008.05.008

[73] Farhoudi B, Alipour A, Ghodrati S, Seyedalinaghi S, Zanganeh M, Mohraz M. "Barriers to adherence to antiretroviral treatment among inmates of a prison in Tehran, Iran: A qualitative study," Archives of. Clinical Infectious Diseases;**13**(2):e57911

[74] Lobato MN et al. Adverse events and treatment completion for latent tuberculosis in jail inmates and homeless persons. Chest. 2005;**127**(4):1296-1303

[75] Davies NECG, Karstaedt AS. Antiretroviral outcomes in South African Prisoners: A retrospective cohort analysis. PLoS ONE;**7**(3):e33309

[76] De Juan J et al. Multicenter study on the discontinuation and efficacy of chronic hepatitis C treatment in the Spanish penitentiary population (EPIBAND study). European Journal of Gastroenterology and Hepatology. 2014;**26**(10):1083-1089

[77] Bock NN, Herron GD, Rogers T, Tapia JR, DeVoe B, Geiter LJ. Acceptability of short-course rifampin and pyrazinamide treatment of latent tuberculosis infection among jail inmates. Chest. 2001;**119**(3):833-837

[78] Palepu A, Tyndall MW, Chan K, Wood E, Montaner JSG, Hogg RS. Initiating highly active antiretroviral therapy and continuity of HIV care: The impact of incarceration and prison release on adherence and HIV treatment outcomes. Antiviral Therapy. 2004;**9**(5):713-719

[79] Seaman SR, Brettle RP, Gore SM. Mortality from overdose among injecting drug users recently released from prison: Database linkage study. British Medical Journal. 1998;**316**(7129):426-428

[80] Stephenson BL, Wohl DA, Golin CE, Tien HC, Stewart P, Kaplan AH. Effect of release from prison and re-incarceration on the viral loads of HIV-infected individuals. Public Health Reports. 2005;**120**(1):84-88

[81] United Nations. United Nations Standard Minimum Rules for the Treatment of Prisoners (the Nelson

Mandela Rules). Vienna: United Nations Office on Drugs and Crime; 2015

[82] Blaauw E, Vermunt R, Kerkhof A. Deaths and medical attention in police custody. Medicine and Law. 1997;**16**(3):593-606

[83] Heide S, Kleiber M, Hanke S, Stiller D. Deaths in German police custody. European Journal of Public Health, Article. 2009;**19**(6):597-601. DOI: 10.1093/eurpub/ckp084

[84] Mills A, Lathlean J, Bressington D, Forrester A, van Veenhuyzen W, Gray R. Prisoners' experiences of antipsychotic medication: Influences on adherence. Journal of Forensic Psychiatry and Psychology, Article. 2011;**22**(1):110-125. DOI: 10.1080/14789949.2010.509804

[85] Stern MF, Greifinger RB, Mellow J. Patient safety: Moving the bar in prison health care standards. American Journal of Public Health. 2010;**100**(11):2103-2110

Chapter 4

Patient Safety in Emergency Medical Services

Bryan R. Wilson and Ashley Woodrow

Abstract

Patients deserve high-quality, evidence-based care delivered from the moment they call for help to the moment they are safely delivered to the hospital. Often patient safety is not viewed as a fun or exciting topic by prehospital clinicians, but it need not be a burden. A culture of safety in emergency medical services can enhance patient outcomes and improve the overall safety in a community. The design and structure of the ambulance are the first layer of protection for patients. Couple that with ambulance operations topics, such as speed and light and siren use and that covers a large swath of the patient safety engineered into the system. There are patient-focused topics such as medication safety protocols, structured handoffs, and competency assessments of high-risk procedures that all serve to increase patient safety. Lastly, an emergency medical services clinician-oriented topic that also heavily impacts our patients is fatigue mitigation. Actively addressing fatigue and employing fatigue mitigation strategies can be used to enhance the safety of patients and will likely enhance the experience of prehospital clinicians in the organization.

Keywords: emergency medical services, EMS, patient safety, medication safety, lights and sirens, EMS vehicle operations, paramedics, fatigue, transfer of care, SBAR, DMIST

1. Introduction

In the landmark document, "EMS Agenda 2050" leaders are challenged to create a people-centered emergency medical services (EMS) system that "serves as the front line of a region's healthcare system and plays a core role in supporting the well-being of community residents and visitors through data-driven, evidence-based, and safe approaches to prevention, response, and clinical care" [1]. While not a new topic in healthcare, the inclusion of safety in this statement represents the first time that the topic is introduced into a federal government publication on emergency medical services, marking the progress and importance of patient safety initiatives. The challenge is many of the interventions that increase safety can be difficult to implement for a number of reasons: cost, resistance to culture change, and a lack of knowledge of the risks involved, just to name a few. So how do we create a system that focuses on the patient first, but also is not wasteful? Can we create a system that takes into consideration the clinician and the patient together? Thankfully, there have been years of research into this question and many national stakeholders have provided resources to help inform our decision-making in this area. Patient safety endeavors not only keep the patient safe but avoiding harm and errors can serve to enhance the well-being of the EMS system workforce, it is a topic that is widely discussed given developing shortages in staffing [2]. The burden that medical errors place on the healthcare system and the economy at large has come into clearer focus since the Institute of Medicine's landmark white paper "To Err is Human." Estimated to cost between $17 and $29 billion in 2000, "preventable adverse events" are a huge burden on the healthcare system, but errors are not the only aspect of the EMS system that focuses on patient safety [3]. As a system of care, there are many aspects of emergency medical services to explore that have an impact on patient safety.

2. Methods

Research pertinent to this manuscript was performed using a comprehensive literature search strategy. Internet-based search platforms used during the preparation of this manuscript included Google™ Scholar, PubMed, and Bioline International. Specific search terms included, but were not limited to, "patient safety," "emergency medical services," "EMS," "medication safety," "medication cross-check," "ambulance safety," "transfer of care," "SBAR," and "stretch operations," out of a total of 5,938,485 initial search results, we narrowed down our reference list to approximately 340 results highly specific to our intended area of focus. Further screened and excluded were sources that did not specifically address the concepts of patient safety in the prehospital environment. After the above screening was completed, our literature sources were narrowed down to the list of 48 citations included herein.

3. Ambulance configuration

One of the first aspects of safety to consider is the design of the ambulance. These vehicles serve their communities by responding to emergency calls and transporting patients to the hospital, so ensuring they operate appropriately and safely is vital to the nation's EMS systems. Whether it is how they are visible to other drivers, how their lights and sirens are configured for emergency responses, how necessary equipment is stored, or how the patient is secured inside the vehicle, there are standards that exist to describe how to safely design an ambulance. These standards are described in detail in this chapter.

While ambulance design and configuration can be viewed as an occupational safety initiative intending to keep our EMS clinicians safe, it also serves as a patient safety consideration as well since these vehicles deliver life-saving care and transport our patients [4, 5]. The absence of an ambulance at a scene or an unnecessary delay can result in worse outcomes for some time-sensitive conditions that the patient is experiencing. Likewise, the patient can be seriously injured inside the ambulance in the event of a crash or stretcher loading mishap. For this reason, aspects of ambulance configuration will be discussed to emphasize their importance for patient safety.

There are 3 main recognized ambulance configuration standards: (1) Federal Specification for Star-of-Life Ambulances (KKK-A-1822(F)) published by the United States General Services Administration; (2) National Fire Protection Agency (NFPA) 1917: Standard for Automotive Ambulances; and (3) Commission on Accreditation of Ambulances Services (CAAS) Ground Vehicle Standards (GVS). These are generally referred to as K-Specs, NFPA 1917, and GVS, respectfully, and this nomenclature will be used in this document. It is important to note the K-specs undergo annual updates posted as separate notices and not attached to the published standard document, whereas the other documents are updated occasionally, and the full published document is updated. This fact makes interpretation and understanding K-spec more difficult than other standards due to the need to review and cross-reference different documents.

While these three organizations publish separate but similar standards, it is rarely up to the individual agency to decide which standard to follow. Since EMS is regulated at the state level, each state decides which standards ambulances must follow. The National Association of State EMS Officials (NASEMSO) developed a project called SafeAmbulances.org through a grant from the National Institute of Standards and Technology (NIST) in 2015 that outlined how different states handle these regulations and provided a background of how each of the backgrounds developed. **Table 1** below shows a breakdown of how many states require each standard in the regulations [6]. It should be noted that CAAS and NFPA have fees associated with their organization and as such, no states require only one of these organization's standards, typically allowing a choice to utilize them if an organization wishes to. GSA K-specs are by far the most popular with over half of the states requiring at least this standard. Lastly, for those states that utilize their own state-specific standards, many employ at least some of the K-spec standards as the foundation [6].

Perhaps the largest change in ambulance safety configuration occurred in 2015 when the GSA adopted a new standard published by the Society of Automobile Engineers (SAE). This new standard, SAE J3027, changed the allowed amount of movement for a stretcher in the event of a frontal impact. Through years of analyzing crash data involving EMS units and creating their own simulated crashes, this organization took steps to make sure that all patients are protected in the event of an ambulance crash [7]. As a result of this change, the old stretcher mounting system was no longer compliant with K-spec standards since the SAE specification is noted in the K-spec standard. At the same time, SAE's new standard also recommended changes to the restraint system on the stretcher itself, which is a huge advancement for the safety of patients as these standards actually considered the varying sizes of the US patient population to ensure ergonomically efficient standards [8]. The pairing of these two changes together ensures that patients, when properly restrained, minimize their risk of injury from dislodgement of the stretcher or breaking free from the restraints.

Nosocomial infections represent a significant burden to the healthcare system, as they are associated with increased mortality, length of stay, and costs [9]. One systematic review identified a high prevalence of organisms, commonly associated with these nosocomial infections [10]. Because of this impact, an important aspect of the design of ambulances is infection prevention. Specifically, all 3 standard-setting organizations have requirements for materials that can and cannot be used inside the vehicle. To prevent cross-contamination between patients, the inside of the ambulances may not contain "absorbent material such as carpeting, fabric, or indoor/outdoor plastic-type

No standard	State specific	GSA K-spec	CAAS GVS	NFPA 1917	Multiple*
4	17	14	0	0	16

**Any combination of GSA, CAAS, and/or NFPA standards totals to 51 as the District of Columbia is included.*

Table 1.
Ambulance safety standards breakdown.

carpeting, that resists cleaning and decontamination" [11]. From the design of the structure to the materials used inside the ambulance, all these complex standards contribute to keeping Americans safe while receiving care inside ambulances.

4. Ambulance operations

The creation of a safe ambulance only goes so far in ensuring the safety of patients. A large onus belongs to the prehospital clinicians caring for the patient. The manner in which a vehicle is operated is paramount to ensure safety features function as designed. Speed, the use of lights and siren warning devices, and positioning of the vehicle at scenes are all things to consider.

4.1 Traffic laws

Many people falsely believe that just because an ambulance has lights and sirens they can ignore traffic laws related to speed, intersection control devices, and passing. That is not the case, however, and emergency vehicle operators should be familiar with their jurisdiction's laws. In New Jersey, for example, there is a statutory requirement that an emergency vehicle must be operated in a manner showing "due regard for the safety of all persons," but ambulances are missing from the "exemption from speed regulations" provision of NJ Code Title 39 [12]. In Pennsylvania, however, ambulances are specifically noted in their motor vehicle code. Per their state law, ambulances are prevented from exceeding speed limits or proceeding through traffic control devices or stop signs until they have come to a full stop and ascertained that they have been given the right of way [13]. All EMS clinicians should review their local rules and regulations to make sure they understand how they are allowed to operate in their jurisdiction. It should be noted, though, that just because an ambulance can operate in a certain manner does not mean that it should. There has been much discussion about improved patient outcomes when prehospital clinicians drive calmly, deliberately, and without speeding as this allows treatments to continue and for minimizing hemodynamic changes that can occur with excessive endogenous epinephrine release [14].

4.2 Emergency warning devices

One of the most serious risks in providing prehospital care is surprisingly not related to medical treatment, but rather how the patient is transported from the scene to the hospital. Though the use of lights and sirens (L&S) decreases response and transport times for just a couple of minutes on average, it increases the risk of ambulance crashes during response by 50% and threefold during patient transport [15]. Despite these statistics, a vast majority of responses and nearly a quarter of patient transports occur using L&S [14]. Not only does this pose a direct threat to the EMS clinicians and patients on board but also can cause delays in patient care, injure the public, ruin expensive essential equipment, and tie up resources that could otherwise be used elsewhere. In a joint position statement released by NAEMSP and various other organizations in 2022, it is advised that "L&S should only be used for situations where the time saved by L&S operations is anticipated to be clinically important to a patient's outcome" [9]. However, there are different factors that must be taken into consideration when discussing which circumstances require L&S in response to a call versus transport to a hospital.

Determination of response priority should be determined by standardized emergency medical dispatch protocols [16]. When writing and implementing these protocols, L&S should be reserved for medical conditions in which a few-minute delay in medical care would be detrimental to the patient's health. Such conditions include significant airway compromise, respiratory and cardiac arrest, loss of consciousness, advanced stages of shock, obstetrical emergencies, and severe trauma. Recent studies have shown these situations to be exceedingly rare [17]. Special exceptions to this standard may be made in situations where significantly delayed response is anticipated due to distance or traffic and the patient has a real potential to decompensate into one of the above categories due to the extended response. In addition to EMD protocols that reflect cautious use of L&S, it is also imperative that dispatchers are properly certified and receive continuing education, which enforces the necessity of keeping priority responses at a safe minimum [14].

Though L&S responses to scenes can be standardized, the utilization of L&S when transporting to the hospital is much less scriptable and statistically more dangerous [14]. When deciding whether or not to utilize L&S, an EMS clinician must quickly evaluate whether or not shortening the transport time by an average of three or four minutes would actually be beneficial [14]. In some cases, such as STEMIs, strokes, and trauma, early notification of the hospital of the impending arrival of the alert allows for advanced preparation leading to improvement in patient outcomes [18]. This time saving may allow for a non-L&S transport, during which the prehospital clinician maximizes medical treatment and stabilization of the condition without the increased risk of being involved in a motor vehicle accident. However, in situations where the patient is rapidly deteriorating or has significant airway compromise, the use of L&S during transport may be warranted. If the use of L&S is unavoidable, there are ways to optimize safety throughout transport.

1. Identifying potential hazards prior to the event: Risk analyses should be performed by EMS agencies to identify potentially hazardous intersections and roadways that increase the risk during an L&S response. EMS clinicians should be made aware of said dangers and avoid them during the L&S transport when possible.

2. Ensure a sterile cockpit: Though not proven, it is thought that the majority of increased risk in an L&S transport is due to driver distraction. Without a second person up front to answer radio communications, manage the control board, and potentially identify road hazards, these duties become additional duties and potential distractions for the emergency vehicle operator. The driver of the emergency vehicle should minimize these distractions and should be familiar with the locations and proper use of all signals, controls, and radios prior to utilizing a vehicle.

3. Emergency vehicle operator training: All emergency vehicle operators should receive rigorous training and continuing education on proper use of an emergency vehicle and should be well versed on the laws and policies pertaining to emergency vehicle operation specific to their state.

4. Agency-wide QA review of L&S use: Agencies should routinely review all transports that require the utilization of L&S and give constructive feedback to their employees on the appropriateness of such.

While this list is not exhaustive, these are some steps that can improve the safety of using lights and sirens. No one step can totally remove the risk involved in L&S use, so agencies are encouraged to take a comprehensive quality improvement approach when it comes to decreasing the use of L&S during transport and response. Each agency needs to weigh the risks and benefits of L&S use and nonuse with other aspects of their system's operation and performance and decide how to proceed. The data are clear though, agencies provide safer care when there is a focus on decreasing the use of L&S, as such every agency should cut their use in some part of their operation [16].

5. Stretcher operations

Though rare, patient injuries from stretcher-related incidents do occur and can pose a significant risk to both the patient and the EMS clinician. In a retrospective study reviewing the 671 reported stretcher-related incidents occurring from 1996–2005, 52 patients were injured, resulting in injuries from lacerations and fractures to traumatic brain injury and death [19]. Not surprisingly, injuries to personnel occurred at a higher rate than to patients, with most of those injuries occurring as sprains/strains. This may seem like an insignificant number of injuries given the 10-year span of data; however, this data is only from incidents reported to the FDA and is likely an underrepresentation of risk. Injuries occurred due to numerous reasons and can be classified into four broad categories: equipment malfunction, operator error, surface conditions, and patient-related [20].

5.1 Equipment malfunction

With the repetitive use of stretchers on patients of varying sizes and over a variety of terrains, it is natural for these to have significant wear and tear over time. Though the breakdown is inevitable, prehospital clinicians should routinely check stretchers to ensure all parts are present and working properly. Any equipment not passing inspection should be immediately taken from the ambulance so that it can be repaired by a qualified professional. It may be inconvenient to take a vehicle out of service over a small missing part or break, but this could potentially lead to a devastating injury from a stretcher failure.

5.2 Operator error

As with all aspects of the job, knowing how to fully operate a piece of equipment safely is imperative, and a stretcher is no exception. Before a patient is ever placed on the stretcher, an operator should be comfortable demonstrating all the functions required for safe use. Partners should also practice lifting, loading, and unloading a stretcher together to ensure development of a systematic approach to ensure proper timing of releases, therefore optimizing safety. In the study by Wang, the largest portion of injuries occurred while unloading the patient from the ambulance [19]. A two-person unloading technique should be utilized to ensure the undercarriage deploys correctly and the stretcher does not collapse. Other potential human errors leading to injury include not latching the stretcher properly into the ambulance safety latch upon loading and not utilizing the recommended safety restraints prior to movement.

5.3 Surface conditions

EMS clinicians work in a variety of environments, regardless of weather conditions. Rain, ice, and snow pose a threat to safety with moving, loading, and unloading stretchers by creating slippery conditions beyond the control of the clinician. These conditions have been shown to precipitate tipping events during movement, as a patient shifting on the mattress in response to slipping or sliding can throw the entire stretcher off balance. In these cases, it may be helpful to have an extra set of hands available to stabilize the side of the stretcher throughout the movement. Additionally, it can be very difficult to safely load and unload a patient when both the stretcher and the floor of the ambulance are covered in precipitation. In these cases, having towels on hand to dry off the floor and the locking mechanism could prove useful in ensuring both patient and crew safety. Though hazards such as cracks in the concrete and uneven gravel surfaces are beyond the control of EMS personnel, keeping a watchful eye for such barriers to safe stretcher use and having a plan for navigating them safely is highly recommended to prevent injury.

5.4 Patient related

The two patient-related stretcher issues most likely to cause harm to the patient and EMS clinician are combative and morbidly obese patients. Combative patients can easily tip a stretcher during movement, therefore, it is important to ensure that the patient is either calmed or appropriately restrained prior to movement. If possible, have extra personnel to secure the sides during movement to prevent tipping. If feasible, it may also be beneficial to walk the patient to the ambulance, securing the patient to the stretcher just prior to loading. Obese patients lend another challenge, not only due to weight and safety harness size limitations of a stretcher but also for crew safety while lifting. Never place more weight on a stretcher than recommended by the manufacturer, as this could lead to catastrophic injuries from collapse, and use safety belt extensions as needed to properly secure the patient to the stretcher. For stretcher lifts and loading of obese patients, maximizing the number of personnel available to help is important for both patient safety and career longevity. Despite typical EMS job descriptions displaying a lifting requirement in the range of 100–200 pounds, the NIOSH recommended load limit set per healthcare clinician is 51 pounds [3]. Surprisingly, the use of hydraulic stretchers does not completely mitigate the risk of injury when lifting an obese patient, as hydraulic stretchers are significantly heavier than manual stretchers [21]. When faced with lifting any type of stretcher with an obese patient, increasing the starting height of the stretcher and ensuring use of proper body mechanics can be advantageous in preventing injury.

6. Medication safety

The five "rights" of medication safety, "right medication, right dose, right patient, right route, and right time" are ingrained in the foundation of every pharmacological safety discussion, yet most medication errors stem from one of these five "rights" being wrong. Medication errors are made even by the most careful and experienced clinicians; therefore, a system of safety checks should be established. Medication errors are rarely simple and typically are complex system failures. Creating a culture of safety around medications can be challenging due to many reasons, such as preconceived notions or workplace rumors. Recently, a medication error made national headlines that resulted in a nurse being charged with and found guilty of criminally negligent homicide [22]. Critics of this decision have all called this action a step back regarding patient safety [23]. Agencies should maintain a comprehensive medication safety policy that encourages reports of events and near-hit events and allows for a root cause analysis to make changes to the system to prevent a recurrence. Outlined below are some ideas and concepts that can be utilized to enhance patient safety when it comes to medication errors.

6.1 Medication cross-checks

Medication cross-checks, or having a second qualified professional verbally verify that the appropriate medication and dose have been selected for the patient's size and condition, have been proven to be effective in preventing most medication errors [24]. During a 54-month period, these authors showed that implementing the system shown in reduced monthly errors from a rate of 0.19 to 0.09%. As opposed to other steps to ensure patient safety, this one is unique as it requires no up-front costs.

Despite the known benefit of cross-checks, they are not always utilized due to high-stress situations, varying levels of partner certifications, the delay when cross-checks are needed for multiple medications, and in administration of medications to pediatric patients. Creating this kind of culture of safety can also be difficult because of stigmas associated with patient safety, which serves as another barrier for implementation of these kinds of systems.

6.2 Pediatric medication safety considerations

In addition to cross-checks, easy-to-read medication aids or checklists, which include indications, contraindications, dosage and administration amount, and route of delivery, could serve as a protective layer against medication errors. These medication aids are especially important in the case of pediatric patients, as weight-based dosing in kilograms is the standard of care and errors in dose calculations are common. According to a position paper released by the NAEMSP in 2020, all pediatric medication aids should list the volumetric amount of a weight-based dose to be given instead of a mass-based amount [25]. For example, a chart referencing pediatric acetaminophen dosing based on the standard concentration of 160mg/5 mL would list that a child weighing 11 kg would receive 5mL of acetaminophen rather than 160 mg. Any changes in formulary concentration should be immediately communicated and medication aids revised to reflect such changes as soon as possible. Another step to take is requiring all weights entered in the ePCR to be in kilograms and not pounds [25]. This is a simple standard to adopt but seeks to eliminate any confusion between pounds and kilograms in the management of patients.

6.3 Medication storage

Safe medication storage is vital to patient safety, and careful consideration must be taken when selecting medications for EMS use and in what arrangement they are kept. When selecting medications, there are many factors that influence what medications should be included in an algorithm. As it pertains to storage, temperature, naming, packaging, varying concentrations, and compatibility requirements should be thoroughly planned out prior to medication selection and storage.

6.4 Temperature

When choosing medications to be included in local EMS protocols, the ability to store a medication at an appropriate temperature is important for both patient safety and cost reduction. For instance, an advanced life support (ALS) crew would typically align protocol medications with what is preferred at the receiving facilities. In the case of benzodiazepines, lorazepam is often preferred for sedation within emergency departments because of the longer half-life and smaller individual dosages. However, this may be impractical for EMS use, as it experiences statistically significant degradation in warmer temperatures and must be replaced every 60 days [26]. For agencies operating in warmer climates, the degradation occurs even faster. Therefore, ambulances in hotter climates must be either stocked with midazolam, which does not degrade in higher temperatures, or have the ability to refrigerate lorazepam appropriately. Unfortunately, temperature degradation can occur with medications across all classes, necessitating cautious choices and strict medication rotation regimens to ensure efficacy. Using a medication with decreased potency or efficacy is certainly not in the best interest of a patient.

6.5 Naming

Medication names can be equally important to patient safety in the selection and storage process. Look-alike and sound-alike medication names are a common source of medication errors, whether due to EMS clinician confusion or grabbing the wrong medication because they were stored in proximity. For example, a paramedic might intend for a patient with stable rapid atrial fibrillation to receive diltiazem, but what if it were stored next to diazepam and was administered instead? Not only would the patient not receive the appropriate medication but it would also become difficult to assess stability of the patient, as they would likely become lethargic and possibly hypotensive due to the adverse effects of the benzodiazepine. In cases where look-alike and sound-alike medications are both part of the EMS protocols, these should be clearly labeled and stored in separate locations [27, 28].

6.6 Packaging

As with look-alike and sound-alike medication names, medications can also be packaged in similar vial sizes or box colors. Ideally, these issues would be engineered out of the system by manufacturers, and in some cases they are. However, there are numerous times when different medications from different manufacturers look similar. When storing medications with similar packaging, try to keep maximum distance between look-alike packages within the medication box. Additionally, agencies should point out these high-risk situations before they become a problem (i.e. when the new packaging is noted, staff should be notified of the similarities before using it with a patient). In the event of a mix-up, medication cross-checks could prevent a medication error due to packaging issues [27, 28].

6.7 Medications with varying concentrations

If possible, avoid procuring varying concentrations of the same medications unless medically necessary. For example, if ketamine was initially purchased at a concentration of 10mg/mL but became unavailable due to supply chain issues, necessitating a switch to a more concentrated 50mg/mL concentration, this could pose a significant threat to patient safety if both concentrations ended up in the same drug box. In order to avoid overdose, it would be appropriate to not only make clinicians aware of the change but also to remove all vials of the more dilute medication from all agency medication boxes. In cases where varying concentrations are necessary, such as in the case of epinephrine, clear labeling, separate storage sites, and medication cross-checks should be employed to prevent medication errors [28].

6.8 Compatibility

Medications that must be diluted prior to administration should be stored together in order to avoid confusion and to ensure the proper diluent or solvent is chosen. For example, amiodarone for infusion should be stored with D5W so that it is not accidentally mixed with an incompatible diluent such as normal saline. Storing medications that must be coadministered in the same location also allows for expedient administration, decreasing the amount of time spent searching for the appropriate concentration or volume of medication or diluent.

7. Transfer of care

Communication skills are crucial for patient safety yet transfer of vital information from EMS clinician to receiving facility personnel is often noted as a source of medical error. It is not only what is communicated between clinicians, but how the information is delivered that affects patient safety. Transfer of care is such a critical juncture for patient safety that in 2013 the National Association of EMS Physicians (NAEMSP) and the American College of Emergency Physicians (ACEP) published a joint physician statement (along with three other key organizations) outlining the importance of this time and highlighting key elements to ensure patient safety when this occurs [29].

7.1 Structured Handoff

In addition to patient demographics, essential information, such as history of present illness, vital signs, interventions, responses to the interventions, and results of any diagnostic testing such as ECG's and point of care laboratory results, should be clearly conveyed to the receiving clinician. In order to prevent information loss in high-acuity situations, a standardized approach to handoff should be developed and routinely used, whether by the EMS clinician or the employing agency itself. There are many different forms of structured handoffs, but two of the more common are SBAR and DMIST (**Table 2**).

7.1.1 SBAR

One such method commonly used by hospitals is the SBAR approach, which is conveying information regarding the situation, background, assessment, and recommendations, in that order, for every handoff and request for evaluation or

SBAR	DMIST
Situation	Demographics
Background	Mechanism
Assessment	Injuries/illness
Recommendations	Signs [Vital Signs]
	Treatments

Table 2.
Structure handoff formats.

intervention. In hospitals, this has been shown to improve safety of patients during handoff [30]. Though this has not been tested in an EMS environment, this can be applied to a patient handoff to maximize patient safety.

1. *Situation:* Who are you providing treatment to and for what? How high is the acuity of this patient's condition? What were you called to the scene for?

   Example: Ms. Smith is a 56-year-old female in significant respiratory distress. Her husband reports that she has asthma and has tried her albuterol inhaler several times today without relief from her symptoms.

2. *Background*: What relevant medical information or prescribed medications are pertinent to the current condition?

   Example: She takes both inhaled corticosteroids and a leukotriene modifier daily and has not missed any doses. She has not required oral steroids for her asthma recently but was intubated 2 years ago for a severe asthma exacerbation.

3. *Assessment*: What were the critical diagnostic or physical exam findings? What interventions were attempted? How effective were they?

   Example: She was found in a tripod position, respiratory rate of 36, SpO2 82% on room air, with both nasal flaring and intercostal retractions, and minimal air movement on lung auscultation. She was given two duonebs and 125mg solumedrol and also placed on supplemental oxygen via nasal cannula, resulting in a slight improvement in SpO2 but no change in respiratory rate, work of breathing, or lung sounds.

4. *Recommendations*: What do you feel are the necessary next steps? EMS providers are encouraged to make recommendations within their respective scope of practice, as an EMS clinician's continued assessments and resulting concerns are helpful in directing immediate care.

   Example: Because of her continued respiratory distress despite nebulizer treatments, steroids, and oxygen administration, I am concerned that she may need further interventions, such as noninvasive positive pressure ventilation or intubation.

7.1.2 DMIST

Another common structured patient handoff technique is the MIST or DMIST tool. Unlike SBAR, where there has not been extensive study of prehospital use, MIST has been studied in multiple centers, including the Southwest Texas Regional Advisory Council, which published one of the largest studies of its use involving over 100 prehospital clinicians pre and post implementation. The overwhelming results of the implementation show that all involved felt that communication between the hospital and prehospital team improved [31]. In 2019, the Commonwealth of Pennsylvania implemented the use of DMIST statewide with a small modification, adding the D for demographics at the beginning [32]. To this point, there has not been comprehensive patient outcome data on this tool.

1. *Demographics*: Age, gender, and weight (as appropriate). This is intended to be simple and for the whole team's knowledge. Information, such as an address, date of birth, and phone number, can be exchanged after transfer of care with hospital registration staff.

2. *Mechanism*: In the trauma setting, this includes time of injury, type of injury, and additional info, such as speed, type of collision, height of fall, type of weapon, and safety devices used. In the medical setting, this includes a review of the *OPQRST* [onset, pain, quality, radiation, severity, and timing].

3. *Injuries/illness*: In the trauma setting, the clinician should list injuries from head to toe. In the medical setting, this includes a review of the SAMPLE history, EKG, Stroke Scale, and other screenings as needed.

4. *Signs (vital signs):* Including GCS, heart rate, blood pressure, respirations, oxygen saturation, and blood sugar.

5. *Treatment*: This is the time when the clinician can review the care provided, such as airway interventions, oxygen delivery, IVs, medications, chest decompression, defibrillators, wound care, splinting, and other interventions. The clinician should also provide relevant patient responses to key interventions.

   Example: This is a 24yo M unrestrained driver frontal impact MVC, car vs tree. He was unconscious at the scene, with an obvious head injury, bruising of the chest wall with crepitus, and bruising of the abdomen. He has obvious lower extremity deformity. His GCS was 3, HR 120, BP 100/50, RR 6, and SATs 80%. He was emergently intubated with no medications for airway protection and his SATs improved to the 90s. He became hypotensive in the 70s following intubation and underwent bilateral chest decompression with an improvement of SpO2 to 100% and BP to 108/62. He has two bilateral 16g IVs in the AC. Received 1000mg TXA at 1002 hours. He received no other medications from us, including any sedative post intubation. We splinted his lower extremity and maintained a cervical collar with c-spine precautions for the duration of the extrication and transport. Any questions?

One part to note about many systems that have implemented the DMIST structured handoff is the "EMS timeout," where the trauma team takes 30 seconds of no action to listen to the EMS clinicians uninterrupted. This time-out can occur upon arrival in the trauma bay while still on the EMS stretcher for the stable patient or after critical interventions have occurred in the unstable trauma patient.

These two examples represent potential methods of content delivery, and it would be perfectly acceptable to formulate alternative handoff communication algorithms, which meet the needs of the individual or EMS agency. Whatever style is adopted, ensure that the skill is practiced and utilized with every patient, and its implementation occurs in partnership with the receiving hospitals. This ensures that in high-stress situations, the report becomes automatic and easy to deliver, without loss of information leading to adverse patient outcomes. Studies continue to show that this is a high-risk area that needs continuous improvement [33].

7.2 Delivery

How information is delivered is just as important as the message content, which is being communicated. Handoff communication should be clear, concise, and without the use of slang or other terminology, which might not be understood by the receiving clinician. Avoid giving handoff during patient transfer from the stretcher to the bed, as the listener may be distracted by the patient's movement and not be actively listening. Ideally, handoff should be given directly to the nurse or physician who will be assuming care, with a verbal demonstration of understanding being given by the receiving clinician (closed-loop communication). A radio report is not considered an adequate handoff, as the receiver will likely not convey all aspects of the report to those who assume care, and important information will likely be lost [29]. Additionally, all critical elements of a verbal handoff should also be documented and available at bedside in case there are questions regarding treatment prior to arrival or if care is transferred to another clinician not present for the initial handoff. Additionally, results of point-of-care testing and copies of the ECG must be made available to the receiving institution so that they may become part of the patient's permanent medical record. A 2009 study found that even in controlled settings, "information gaps" occurred leading to the suggestion that further scrutiny is needed to assess and improve delivery and handoff of information [34].

8. Fatigue

A simple internet search for motor vehicle accidents involving drivers who fell asleep at the wheel yields multiple results of devastating incidents, also populating numerous articles related to first responders being found sleeping on the job. When identifying risks to patient safety, the first things to come to mind are medication errors, high-risk procedures, and equipment malfunctions-issues, which can be mitigated with medication cross-checks, education, safety checklists, and preventive maintenance checks and services. However, according to the World Health Organization, healthcare worker fatigue is the largest contributing factor to both patient injury and medical errors [35]. Fatigue, whether physical or mental, can lead to many threats to patient safety, including delayed judgment making, medication administration errors, slow response to threats or obstacles, and failure to adhere to written protocol. Though inherent to the nature of the job, creation of evidence-based fatigue mitigation programs should be prioritized for both patient and prehospital clinician safety. A strong program should consider the needs of the community, available resources, and clinician feedback, while also incorporating formal education on effects of fatigue and strategies to reduce risk.

8.1 Needs of the community and available resources

When thinking about factors contributing to fatigue, shift length and call volume immediately come to mind. Though it would make sense that the longer an employee works, the more likely they are to be fatigued, available literature suggests that there is no statistically significant difference in the number of unfavorable events, which occur in shifts of varying lengths as long as they are 24 hours or less in duration [35]. This may not make sense at first glance, but it is thought that this could be attributed to the ability to rest between calls and longer periods of time between shifts for those who work 24-hour shifts, which reduces the risk of adverse events. In other healthcare fields, higher individual workload has also been shown to contribute to increased adverse patient events due to effects of fatigue, however, no prehospital studies have been conducted [35, 36]. Regardless, factors such as call volume, transport times, and call acuity should be taken into account prior to determining appropriate shift length to remedy fatigue. However, adjustments to shift structure may not be possible in all response areas given increased costs of additional equipment and lack of available EMS professionals, therefore, other mitigation techniques may be more feasible.

8.2 Clinician feedback

Risks for potential harm due to fatigue cannot be adequately assessed without ongoing structured feedback from those in the field. Knowing how fatigued EMS clinicians feel, what resources would be valued for combatting fatigue, and how the fatigue is affecting both their personal and professional lives is crucial in tailoring both educational programs and risk-reduction tools to the needs of the individual agency. No validated assessment survey is currently available; however, this should not prevent an agency from seeking such information [37].

8.3 Education

How can EMS personnel know the seriousness of fatigue and how to prevent those poor personal and patient outcomes if the topic is never formally addressed? Routine education covering topics such as sleep disorders, successful sleep habits, health maintenance, and circadian rhythm awareness could be beneficial [37]. Additionally, clinicians should be educated on the mitigation techniques employed by an agency and available resources that may be utilized. Continuing education on the topic also opens the door for further dialogue, enhancing the quality and quantity of the feedback necessary to develop risk reduction strategies in the first place.

8.4 Formal guidelines about fatigue in EMS

In response to numerous research projects demonstrating the negative impacts of fatigue on patient safety, the National Association of State EMS Officials, in conjunction with the National Highway Traffic Safety Administration (NHTSA), published a set of five evidence-based guidelines in 2017 [37]. Though each guideline may not be universally applicable given the individual needs of a community or EMS organization, it does set the framework for agencies to establish their own system of fatigue hazard mitigation (**Table 3**).

These recommendations serve as a tool but not a comprehensive list of innovative strategies to decrease risks to patient safety due to EMS clinician fatigue. It remains the responsibility of an agency to conduct its own internal assessment of practitioner

Recommendation	Strength of recommendation	Quality of evidence
Use fatigue/sleepiness survey instruments to measure and monitor fatigue in EMS personnel	Strong	Low
Recommend that EMS personnel work shifts shorter than 24 hours in duration	Weak	Very low
Recommend that EMS personnel have access to caffeine as a fatigue countermeasure	Weak	Low
Recommend that EMS personnel have the opportunity to nap while on duty to mitigate fatigue	Weak	Very low
Recommend that EMS personnel receive education and training to mitigate fatigue and fatigue-related risks	Weak	Low

Table 3.
Evidence-based fatigue management recommendations.

fatigue, develop mitigation techniques unique to its service, and reassess the practicality and effectiveness of these policies [38]. Ultimately, regardless of shift length or agency guidelines, an EMS professional should develop their own personal health and sleep regimen to prevent fatigue to avoid making critical mistakes or the news headlines for an adverse event.

9. High-risk procedures

When reading through NHTSA's "National Scope of EMS Model," some of the more notable complex procedures within the paramedic's minimum psychomotor skill set include intubation, decompression of the pleural space, and percutaneous cricothyrotomy [39]. It is important to clarify that these are minimums, and the potential for even riskier procedures, such as rapid sequence intubation using paralytics, finger thoracostomy, and surgical cricothyrotomy, could be included in an ALS clinician's scope at the discretion of the individual state and agency medical director. These procedures, along with other procedures within the ALS scope of practice, are inherent of higher risk because they require a higher level of understanding of anatomy and physiology, are performed infrequently, require both more initial and continuing education, and come with significant risk to the patient if improperly performed [39]. To improve patient outcomes and decrease risk, adjuncts such as checklists, procedural competency assessments, and clinical simulations should be taken into consideration for inclusion into agency performance improvement algorithms.

9.1 Checklists

Use of procedural checklists to enhance safety has been proven to be effective in various industries, and healthcare is no exception [40]. These point-of-care cognitive aids are a useful way to augment procedural memory and could be especially useful in high-risk prehospital procedures in distracting and austere environments. For example, checklists for intubation have been extensively studied for in-hospital use, and though not proven to have a mortality benefit, checklist use was associated with statistically significant decreases in peri-intubation hypoxic events [41]. One longitudinal before and after a study conducted using data from an air ambulance company concluded that not only did use of checklists decrease hypoxic and hypotensive events during RSI but also improved the first-pass intubation success rates [42]. A similar study on a ground ALS service showed a checklist as part of a bundle of care showed lower rates of peri-intubation hypoxia, further demonstrating that checklists are a helpful resource for patient safety [43].

Though not studied, checklists could be of benefit for improving outcomes in a variety of high-risk prehospital procedures. A high-quality checklist should be easy to read, written in plain language, and could include various data such as patient considerations, necessary equipment and medications, procedural steps, and countermeasures should complications be encountered.

9.2 Competency assessments

Ensuring provider competency prior to performing high-risk procedures is vital to patient safety. Competency assessments should not only be aimed at procedural steps but also include evaluation of appropriateness of use of the high-risk procedure based on patient condition. Just as in medication safety, knowing the indications, alternatives, and ideal patient demographic for a procedure is just as important as being able to physically perform the procedure itself. Initial provider certification is issued based on a basic level of competency to appropriately implement and perform a procedure; however, it is up to an agency to credential a provider based on an assessment of those procedural competencies. In addition to initial credentialing, the NAEMSP recommends that "reverification of a provider's cognitive, affective, psychomotor, and critical thinking skills, pertinent to relevant clinical situations, occurs no less frequently than every two (2) years" [44].

9.3 Simulation

Simulation has been proven effective for evaluating and teaching psychomotor skills, communication, teamwork, and patient management in a variety of medical environments. Though not well studied for use in the prehospital setting, the ability to repeat uncommon, high-risk procedures in a controlled environment affords the provider opportunity to gain experience, education, and muscle memory in tandem [45]. Moreover, prehospital simulations and assessments can be used to strengthen non-procedural skills, such as communication, leadership skills, stress management, and decision-making, all of which are fundamental to patient safety. Simulation is not only useful for initial and ongoing education but also as a remediation tool for both self-identified and agency-specific performance improvement initiatives [46].

10. Conclusion

Patient safety is a complex topic that has to overcome significant resistance to change. Over twenty years since the publication of "To Err is Human," medical adverse events still represent a significant burden to our healthcare system [47]. As discussed above, there are many intricate parts of the system to consider. In some areas, progress has been made, such as engineering safe ambulances and storage compartments. In other areas, such as handoffs, much work is still to be done. In some areas, such as L&S use, there are national partnerships that are seeking to improve systems across the country [48]. The journey to a safer system for our patients will take time, which is why the EMS Agenda 2050 lays out a foundation for improvements to be made over the next 30 years. Partnerships with public safety, public health, healthcare systems, insurers, and the government are necessary to continue growing EMS to fill the need that exists and allow it to develop with these safety mechanisms engrained in the culture. Continued work is needed, but the foundation is strong to create a safer system for patients.

Acknowledgements

The authors wish to acknowledge the contributions of Dr. Dawn Brown who provided valuable ideas and feedback during the development of this text. Inspiration for this text came from the NAEMSP Quality and Safety Course and the NEMSQA National Lights and Siren Collaborative. Funding for open-source publishing was provided by St. Luke's University Health Network's Graduate Medical Education Fund.

Conflict of interest

The authors declare no conflict of interest.

Note and thanks/other

The authors wish to thank the men and women serving in EMS systems across the globe. Without their hard work and dedication, many few lives would be saved——be safe out there.

Author details

Bryan R. Wilson[1*] and Ashley Woodrow[2]

1 St. Luke's University Health Network, Bethlehem, PA, USA

2 St. Luke's Anderson Emergency Medicine Residency, Easton, PA, USA

*Address all correspondence to: bryan.wilson@sluhn.org

References

[1] EMS Agenda 2050 Technical Expert Panel. EMS Agenda 2050: A People-Centered Vision for the Future of Emergency Medical Services (Report No. DOT HS 812 664). Washington, DC: National Highway Traffic Safety Administration; 2019

[2] George K, Sweeny S. State Actions to Address EMS Workforce Shortages. National Conference of State Legislatures [Internet]. 2022. Available from: https://www.ncsl.org/research/health/state-actions-to-address-ems-workforce-shortages.aspx [Accessed: October 10, 2022]

[3] Institute of Medicine (US) Committee on Quality of Health Care in America. In: Kohn LT, Corrigan JM, Donaldson MS, editors. To Err is Human: Building a Safer Health System. Washington (DC): National Academies Press (US); 2000

[4] Centers for Disease Control and Prevention. Emergency Medical Services—NIOSH—CDC [Internet]. 2022. Available from: https://www.cdc.gov/niosh/topics/ems/default.html [Accessed: August 1, 2022]

[5] Ambulance Patient Compartment Human Factors Design Guidebook. US Department of Homeland Security. 2015. Available from: https://www.dhs.gov/sites/default/files/publications/Ambulance%20Patient%20Compartment%20Human%20Factors%20Design%20Guidebook.pdf

[6] National Association of State EMS Officials. SafeAmbulances. [Internet]. 2019. Available from: http:safeambulances.org [Accessed: August 1, 2022]

[7] Castillo D, Bobick T, Pratt S. New Research and Findings from the NIOSH Division of Safety Research. Washington (DC): American Society of Safety Engineers; 2013

[8] Centers for Disease Control and Prevention. Emergency Medical Services—NIOSH—CDC [Internet]. 2022. Available from: https://www.cdc.gov/niosh/topics/ems/data.html [Accessed: September 10, 2022]

[9] Stone PW. Economic burden of healthcare-associated infections: An American perspective. Expert Review of Pharmacoeconomics & Outcomes Research. 2009;**9**(5):417-422

[10] Obenza A, Cruz P, Buttner M, Woodard D. Microbial contamination on ambulance surfaces: a systematic literature review. The Journal of Hospital Infection. 2022;**122**:44-59

[11] US General Services Administration. KKK-A-1822F: Federal Specification for the Star-of-Life Ambulance. 2007. Available from: https://www.ok.gov/health2/documents/KKK-A-1822F%20%2007.01.2007.pdf

[12] New Jersey Revised Statutes. Title 39 - MOTOR VEHICLES AND TRAFFIC REGULATION. Section 39:4-103 [Internet]. Trenton (NJ): State of New Jersey Department of State; 2013. Available from: https://law.justia.com/codes/new-jersey/2013/title-39/section-39-4-103 [cited 2022 Sept 1]

[13] Title 75 PA Motor Vehicle Code. Part III. Section 31A:3501. Harrisburg (PA): Department of Transportation. Available from: https://www.legis.state.pa.us/WU01/LI/LI/CT/HTM/75/00.031..HTM [cited 2022 Sept 1]

[14] Kupas DF. Lights and siren use by emergency medical services: Above all,

do no harm. National Highway Traffic Safety Administration. 2017. Available from: https://www.ems.gov/pdf/Lights_and_Sirens_Use_by_EMS_May_2017.pdf

[15] Watanabe BL, Patterson GS, Kempema JM, Magailanes O, Brown LH. Is use of warning lights and sirens associated with increased risk of ambulance crashes? A contemporary analysis using national EMS information system (NEMSIS) data. Annals of Emergency Medicine. 2019;**74**(1):101-109

[16] Kupas DF, Zavadsky M, Burton B, Baird S, Clawson JJ, et al. Joint statement on lights & siren vehicle operations on emergency medical services responses. Prehospital Emergency Care. 2022;**26**(3):459-461

[17] Jarvis JL, Hamilton V, Taigman M, Brown LH. Using red lights and sirens for emergency ambulance response: How often are potentially life-saving interventions performed? Prehospital Emergency Care. 2021;**25**(4):549-555

[18] Lim CB, Peterson ED, Smith EE, Saver JF, Liang L, Xian Y, et al. Emergency medical service hospital prenotification is associated with improved evaluation and treatment of acute ischemic stroke. Circulation. 2012;**5**:514-522

[19] Wang HE, Weaver MD, Abo BN, Kaliappan R, Fairbanks RJ. Ambulance stretcher adverse events. Quality & Safety in Health Care. 2009;**18**:213-216

[20] Goodloe JM, Crowder CJ, Arthur AO, Thomas SH. EMS stretcher "Misadventures" in a large, urban EMS system: A descriptive analysis of contributing factors and resultant injuries. Emerging Medical International. 2012;**2012**:45706

[21] Prairie J, Plamondon A. Hegg0Deloye S, Larouche D, Corbeil P. Biomechanical risk assessment during field loading of hydraulic stretchers into ambulances. International Journal of Industrial Ergonomics. 2016;**54**:1-9

[22] Timms M. Ex-Nurse RaDonda Vaught Found Guilty on Two Charges in Death of Patient [Internet]. Nashville, TN: The Tennessean; 2022. Available from: https://www.tennessean.com/story/news/crime/2022/03/25/radonda-vaught-trial-vanderbilt-nurse-jury-verdict/7154135001/ [Accessed: August 10, 2022]

[23] Bean M. A backward step for patient safety': Medical groups respond to RaDonda Vaught sentencing. Becker's Hospital Review [Internet]. 2022. Available from: https://www.beckershospitalreview.com/patient-safety-outcomes/a-backward-step-for-patient-safety-medical-groups-respond-to-radonda-vaught-sentencing.html

[24] Misasi P, Keeble JR. Medication safety in emergency medical services: approaching an evidence-based method of verification to reduce errors. Therapeutic Advanced Drug Safety. 2019;**10**:1-14

[25] Cicero MX, Adelgais K, Hoyle JD, Lyng JW, Harris M, Moore B, et al. Medication dosing safety for pediatric patients: recognizing gaps, safety threats, and best practices in the emergency medical services setting. A Position Statement and Resource Document from NAEMSP. Prehospital Emergency Care. 2021;**25**(2):294-306

[26] McMullan JF, Pinnawin A, Jones E, Denninghoff K, Siewart N, et al. The 60-day temperature-dependent degradation of Midazolam and Lorazepam in the prehospital environment. Prehospital Emergency Care. 2013;**17**:1-7

[27] Kupas DF, Shayhorn MA, Green P, Payton TF. Structured inspection of medications carried and stored by

emergency medical services agencies identifies practices that may lead to medication errors. Prehospital Emergency Care. 2012;**16**:67-75

[28] Walker D, Moloney C, SueSee B, Sharples R, Blackman R, Long D, et al. Factors influencing medication errors in the prehospital paramedic environment: A mixed method systematic review. Prehospital Emergency Care. 2022. DOI: 10.1080/10903127.2022.2068089

[29] Transfer of patient care between EMS providers and receiving facilities. Prehospital Emergency Care. 2014;**18**:305-305

[30] De Meester K, Verspuy M, Monsieurs KG, Bogaert PV. SBAR improves nurse-physician communication and reduces unexpected death: A pre and post intervention study. Resuscitation. 2013;**84**:1192-1196

[31] Maddry JK, Simon EM, Reeves LK, Mora AG, Clemons MA, et al. Impact of a standardized patient hand-off tool on communication between emergency medical services personnel and emergency department staff. Prehospital Emergency Care. 2021;**25**:530-538

[32] DMIST. Standardizing the EMS to Trauma Team Patient Handoff in Pennsylvania. 2014. Available from: https://pehsc.org/wp-content/uploads/2014/05/PA-DMIST-PPT.pdf

[33] Goldberg SA, Porat A, Strother CG, Lim NQ, Wijeratne HRS, Sanchez G, et al. Quantitative analysis of the content of EMS handoff of critically ill and injured patients to the emergency department. Prehospital Emergency Care. 2007;**21**:14-17

[34] Carter AJE, Davis KA, Evans LV, Cone DC. Information loss in emergency medical services handover of trauma patients. Prehospital Emergency Care. 2009;**13**:280-285

[35] Patterson PD, Weaver MD, Frank RC, Warner CW, Martin-Gill C, et al. Association between poor sleep, fatigue, and safety outcomes in emergency medical services providers. Prehospital Emergency Care. 2012;**16**:86-97

[36] Patterson PD, Weaver MD, Hostler D, Guyette FX, Callaway CW, Yealy DM. The shift length, fatigue, and safety conundrum in EMS. Prehospital Emergency Care. 2012;**16**:572-576

[37] Patterson PD, Higgins JS, Van Dongen HPA, Buysse DJ, Thackery RW, et al. Evidence-based guidelines for fatigue risk management in emergency medical services. Prehospital Emergency Care. 2018;**22**:89-101

[38] Martin-Gill C, Higgins JS, Van Dongen HPA, Buysse DJ, Thackery RW, et al. Proposed performance measures and strategies for implementation of the fatigue risk management guidelines for emergency medical services. Prehospital Emergency Care. 2018;**22**:102-109

[39] National Association of State EMS Officials. National EMS Scope of Practice Model (Report No. DOT HS 812-666). Washington, DC: National Highway Traffic Safety Administration; 2019

[40] Chen C, Kan T, Li S, Qiu C, Gui L. Use and implementation of standard operating procedures and checklists in Prehospital Emergency Medicine: A literature review. The American Journal of Emergency Medicine. 2016;**34**(12):2432-2439

[41] Turner JS, Bucca AW, Propst SL, Ellender TJ, Sarmiento EJ, et al. Association of checklist use in endotracheal intubation with clinically important outcomes: A Systematic

Review and Met-analysis. JAMA Network Open. 2020;**3**(7):e209278

[42] Weir WB, Olvera D, Lauria M, Noce J. Implementation of a rapid sequence intubation checklist improves first pass success and reduces peri-intubation hypoxia in Critical Care Transport. Air Medical Journal. 2022;**41**(1):24

[43] Jarvis JL, Gonzales J, Johns D, Sager L. Implementation of a clinical bundle to reduce out-of-hospital peri-intubation hypoxia. Annals of Emergency Medicine. 2018;**72**(3):272-279

[44] Clinical credentialing of EMS providers. Prehospital Emerging Care. 2017;**21**(3):397-398

[45] Abelsson A, Rystedt I, Suserud B-O, Lindwall L. Mapping the use of simulation in Prehospital Care—A literature review. Scandinavian Journal of Trauma, Resuscitation and Emergency Medicine. 2014;**22**(1):1-12

[46] Langdalen H, Abrahamsen EB, Sollid SJ, Sørskår LI, Abrahamsen HB. A comparative study on the frequency of simulation-based training and assessment of non-technical skills in the Norwegian Ground Ambulance Services and helicopter emergency medical services. BMC Health Services Research. 2018;**18**(1):509

[47] Bates DW, Singh H. Two decades since to err is human: an assessment of progress and emerging priorities in patient safety. Health Affairs (Millwood). 2018;**37**(11):1736-1743

[48] Lights and Sirens Collaborative. National EMS Quality Alliance [Internet]. 2021. Available from: https://www.nemsqa.org/lights-and-siren

Chapter 5

Emergency Department Restraint Safety

Abby White and Christopher Kustera

Abstract

Restraint use during patient care is a serious and important safety topic because it is often utilized in high stress, rapidly evolving, and unique situations in which patients not only pose harm to themselves, but harm to others. The scope of patient safety topic is a threefold approach: initiation, maintenance, and discontinuation. First, a briefly literature pertaining to evidence-based criteria for the initiation of patient restraints will be constructed. Secondly, restraint types and the resources required to maintain restraints will be explicated. Finally, the chapter will conclude with patient evaluation methods pertaining to the safe discontinuation of restraints and resource de-escalation. A succinct, pragmatic discussion on restraint utilization - a method that mitigates a patient's threat to themselves and others – will be presented in this manuscript.

Keywords: restraints, patient safety, health provider safety, hospital staff safety, agitation, resource management

1. Introduction

Restraint use during patient care is a serious and important safety topic because restraints are often utilized in high stress, rapidly evolving, and unique situations where patients may pose harm to themselves and others. There are a panoply of reasons for the initiation and maintenance of physical and chemical restraints that can range from the protection of patients from self-extubation in the ICU [1] to the prevention of bodily harm and property damage during acute behavioral disturbances (ABDs) in the emergency department (ED) [2–6]. Current restraint literature contains a wide range of studies with varying levels of evidence. Due to this wide range of studies, the proper time to use restraints, the most effective types of restraints, and the proper management of agitated patients is an area of continual research. However, a troubling trend is present upon review of restraint literature – patient aggression in the healthcare sector is increasing [2, 7–13].

An increase in patient aggression is correlated with increased staff turnover and increased "burnout" in EDs [2, 8]. When evaluating United States ED visits, agitation incidence was reported at 2.6% of all visits [14]. A provider must have a plan to address and manage the agitated patient. Therefore, issues regarding restraint utilization are a commonplace challenge in the ED given the wide range and continual change in patient populations [5, 15, 16]. However, why are agitated and violent presentations so prevalent and trending upward? This manuscript will discuss two major factors pertinent to this restraint utilization question.

First, patients commonly access the ED pragmatically to receive *rapid* medical attention as opposed to *emergent* medical care [13]. The twenty-four hour availability of medical attention in the ED has led to increasing ED visits. There is often a disconnect between the expectations of patients-families when compared to health care professional expectations [13]. This cognitive disconnect can develop an environment ripe for "misunderstanding and conflict" [13]. Within a setting of high patient volumes, cramped working areas, mental fatigue, and insufficient administrative support, the addition of areas ripe for misunderstanding place further stress on an already stressed system. Considering this combination of potential patient-provider disconnect and a milieu of onerous situational variables, an already depleted health care workforce continues to suffer from decreased staffing numbers and dangerous lack of resource availability [11, 13]. It is imperative that health care providers have plans and resources in place in order to address situations that could involve violence, assault, and aggression.

Secondly, the increasing prevalence of psychiatric patients with acute behavioral needs provides an increasing level of complexity to the ED workflow. The World Health Organization (WHO) lists psychiatric disorders as "a major impact on health, society, human rights, and economy" while attributing 14% of global disease burden to psychiatric disorders [13]. Psychiatric patients also possess a higher frequency of ED utilization when compared to non-psychiatric patients [9, 13]. Additionally, one of the main reasons for a patient with psychiatric needs to pursue medical attention is violent behavior and incidence of violent behavior is higher in this increased in this population [13]. Therefore, the ED is often a setting where management of acute psychiatric needs are acutely addressed at times of crisis [17]. These acutely agitated patients require additional considerations and resources from staff to address de-escalation, chemical sedation, prevention of elopement, and violence [13]. In a high speed environment with rapid care, health care professionals express difficulty assessing and addressing the needs of this patient population [13]. This challenging communication difficulty provides yet another area for potential development of violent behavior. Naturally, the discussion of restraint use is more frequent in this dangerous setting.

The cumulative effect of incongruence between staff and patient expectations, the utilization of the ED as a primary source of acute behavioral health crisis evaluation, and increasing ABDs makes the ED rife for conflict and agitation. This scenario begets a need for a streamlined processes to provide safety measures for both patients and staff. Restraints are an important but high-risk tool in the management of the agitated patient. Providers must consider the use of this intervention alongside potential complications much like any procedure or medicine. Therefore, both the patient and health care professional perspectives must be considered when contemplating the risks of restraint initiation.

From the perspective of the patients, it is important to consider the risks and factors that lead up to the consideration of restraint initiation. Patient perception and experience in the ED when restraints have been utilized have been studied, and the utilization of restraints has been shown to cause lasting emotional damage to the patient despite a focus on the patient's best interests [9, 14]. This damage can impact the course of their medical care. The therapeutic alliance is often based on the establishment of rapport, a task that is often daunting given the dynamic nature of ED interactions and the challenges of first-time patient introductions. In addition, commonly reported adverse events associated with restraint use are prolonged physical injuries and cardiac events [14].

Verbal de-escalation is an effective mitigating technique, but the ED environment is a challenging setting that may hamper its effectiveness. It is difficult to gain insight to a patient's wants, desires, and goals in the setting of agitation which only further impairs the utilization of verbal de-escalation techniques [14]. With the potential mitigation of verbal de-escalation techniques, difficulty at establishing a de novo therapeutic alliance, and potential adverse reactions to restraints, patients have expressed feeling of coercion and entrapment when restraints are employed [14, 17–20]. While several barriers to de-escalation exist in the ED, frequent failed attempts at de-escalation and increased ED ABDs leads to challenging encounters and the likelihood of restraint placement.

From the perspective of the health care professionals, patient and staff safety is the ultimate goal. This goal can be difficult to obtain. The occurrence of ABDs not only impacts patient's health and management but impacts the health and safety of the staff providing care. A UK study reported that greater than 30% of health care providers reported assault while working with patients in the ED [2]. This number is likely to be grossly underestimated given the total high prevalence of underreporting [2]. The ED has been reported to be one of a medical settings with the "highest risk" of harm [11]. Rates of aggression and assault have been noted to be skewed towards nurses and health-care assistants when compared to all ED personnel [3, 11–13, 21].

2. Methods

A comprehensive literature search was conducted for the creation of this manuscript. Internet-based search platforms used during the preparation of this manuscript included PubMed Central and Scopus. Search terms were: "restraints", "physical restraints", "chemical restraints", "agitation", "emergency departments AND restraints", and "emergency departments AND aggression". Summation of search results totaled 298,534 manuscripts. The references were then limited to publications within the last twenty years. Upon review of this subsect of search results, the reference list was narrowed to 100 documents. These 100 documents were assessed on their relevance to restraint utilization in the ED. These 100 were then assessed on how closely the documents evaluated the management of acutely agitated patients with regards to restraint initiation, management, and discontinuation in the ED. After this final screening, 37 sources were utilized for the construction of this manuscript.

3. Pre-initiation considerations regarding patient restraints

When considering the initiation of patient restraints, the goal is always to control the situation without the initiation of restraints. Many variables and factors can be involved in the situations that precede and evolve into ABDs. These variables can include environmental/architectural factors, hospital policy factors, and practice-based interventions. Most broadly, these variables reside within two major buckets of consideration: proactive vs. reactive measures [11]. This section will parse common listed proactive and reactive measures that can provide potential areas of conflict mitigation to limit or eliminate the need for restraints.

Proactive approaches are important interventions that can potentially stop ABDs before they occur. The literature lists many examples, but they are often discussed in the context of weak to moderate evidence [2, 11, 22]. Although there are many efforts to stop ABDs, no single proactive measure has been able to definitively address ABDs [2, 11]. Without one agreed effective measure, it is then important to review multiple common interventions that are frequently discussed in the literature.

One proactive measure is providing maximum patient visibility in scenarios that include potentially agitated patients [11]. Increased patient visibility by providers can be achieved from a host of interventions. Closed circuit TV (CCTV) and reinforced glassed areas are two common architectural interventions that aid in maximizing visibility. The utilization of increased visibility allows providers to more rapidly identify situations where patients could become agitated (pacing, aggressive verbalizations, responding to inappropriate stimuli, etc.). This could help providers intervene earlier and assess patient needs before the situation evolves to a situation where restraints could be needed. This visibility can also be augmented through the utilization of alarm systems which provide an environmental tool for the management and assessment of patients by providing indications for those who are potentially ambulating or disregarding reorientation methods by staff.

Designated evaluation spaces are another proactive approach towards mitigation and minimization of ABDs. These rooms have been referred to as safe rooms, seclusion areas, and low stimulus environments [2, 11]. They provide modifiable and controllable environments that remove agents that increase agitation, help foster a therapeutic alliance, and increase rapport with patients. In accordance with multiple sources that also include the National Institutes for Care and Excellence (NICE) criteria, there are recommendations regarding the layout of the room that will help with health assessment interviews [2, 11, 23]. The rooms should be as close as possible to the receiving area of the ED [2, 11, 23]. Spacing should also accommodate up to six people and be fitted with technology and windows that help with the ability to observe individuals [2, 11, 23]. This area should also contain furnishing that are soft, be well-ventilated, and contain no items that could be potential utilized as a potential weapon [2, 11, 23]. With some of these variables established, the rooms provide an area that can both mitigate and anticipate of situations involving agitation.

From the purview of practice-based interventions, the utilization of targeted triage screening scales that have been utilized in Psychiatric care have yet to be widely adopted in the ED setting. These triage tools have been identified as a potential area of practice-based intervention [17]. For example, screening questionnaires for proper triaging of individuals experiencing psychosis have been validate in the inpatient settings, but a standardized screening tool regarding psychosis has not been validated in an ED setting [17]. These tools may better identify organic causes of agitation. If one can identify a primary psychiatric cause of agitation as opposed to substance intoxication, better patient triage can prevent escalation to restraint application and provide a clearer view of the incidence and prevalence of ABD presentations in the ED.

Policy interventions targeted towards patient perceptions and timely dissemination of information have also been noted to help mitigate patient agitation occurrences while also improving reported patient experiences [9]. For example, one area of negative patient experience is the perception of "judgmental attitudes" by either staff, EMS, or police present during evaluation [9]. Policy interventions that inform groups of their impact on patient experience are areas that could eliminate behaviors that negatively shape patient agitation. Long wait times also provide situations in which individuals become more agitated. This agitation is alleviated when patients were provided with timely support and information on wait times [2, 11]. Patients also express "vulnerability" and "overstimulation" when ABDs are recorded, so providing areas of privacy and personal space have also been associated with significant improvements to patient reported outcomes and agitation occurrence [9, 14]. Patients express that the use of seclusion and restraint were also mitigated when an advocate who could explain interventions and evaluations was present. These are a sample of policy interventions that can be proactively enacted to mitigate scenarios in which feelings of agitation or aggression could flourish [9].

An additional proactive measure is the implementation of training programs for staff. These training programs can help better train providers in verbal de-escalation techniques and evaluation methods. These training programs have been evaluated to increase provider confidence in addressing ABDs [2, 11]. The number, quality, and names of training programs are too varied and extensive to innumerate within this chapter, so general principles of these programs will be discussed instead. The core competencies of workplace policy knowledge, behavioral theories and aggression etiologies, identification of high risk scenarios, assertiveness, and communication techniques are central to these training programs [11]. Although these programs were associated with increased in ABD interaction confidence, it is important not to conflate confidence with efficaciousness when dealing with ABDs [11]. These training programs do provide another avenue of implementation of tools to help health care professionals with identification of agitation in a quick and efficient way and provide another layer of conflict resolution that can possibly reduce occurrence of ABDs.

Secondly, consider more reactive approaches. These approaches include mobilization of designated teams with the expressed intent of mitigating or addressing the concerns of the agitated patient [11, 19, 24–26]. These resources contain many institution specific naming conventions and personnel classifications that would be outside of the ability of this chapter to fully enumerate, but there are generalizable concepts that occur across these teams. These teams consist of multi-disciplinary teams from a host of backgrounds – administration, security, and nursing to name a few. These teams have designated roles that range from interaction with the patient, interaction with bystanders, interaction with the environment, and interaction with medications and tools. With a clear division of labor and rehearsed practice in these roles, these teams help to specifically address unique clinical scenarios and best mitigate ABDs short of needing to escalate the level of care [2, 11].

The mobilization of security or law enforcement personnel is another resource providers can mobilize during ABDs. It is important to foster relationships with these personnel as they can be invaluable in providing support to mitigate aggressive behavior. However, it is important to note that the presence of law enforcement or security can potentially be a "double-edged sword." For acutely agitated patients, the presence of these support individuals can provide a negative stimulus and may strain the therapeutic alliance if they have had negative interactions with these personnel in the past [20, 27]. Evaluate each patient's situation with regards to each patient's personal history and presenting complaints.

A trained crisis worker or psychiatric emergency services (PES) is an additional area of support and reactive mitigating approaches [17]. These providers have training in acute management and mitigation techniques that are targeted to address agitation secondary to psychiatric disturbances. A variety of techniques, agitation scoring systems, and clinical triaging tools are present and discussed in the psychiatric literature which allows providers to assess developing and established situations [4, 18, 19, 21, 28–30]. These providers can provide additional support and techniques to properly engage with the patient, better assess the source of their agitation, and provide recommendations on further therapy or medication. However, it is important to note that these clinical tools and evaluation techniques are not always validated or easily applicable to the ED setting when compared to inpatient hospital settings. Additionally, not all EDs have access to these providers, and these providers are rarely available twenty-four hours a day. However when present, the utilization of counselors trained in emergency psychiatric services and evaluation reduces the use of restraint and seclusion in cases of psychosis while bolstering a therapeutic alliance [17].

4. Initiation of patient restraints

When environmental/architectural, procedural, and practice-based interventions have been inadequate in staving off agitation and the individual in question has become combative and a threat to staff and self, it is then time to escalate care to the utilization of restraints. Much like the previous section, restraints can be divided into multiple categories: chemical, physical, environmental, and seclusion [22]. Although both chemical and physical restraint are far more commonly discussed in the literature, the utilization of seclusion and the environment as restraint are also important to discuss. Environmental restraint is predominantly the utilization of the items such as fences, walls, doors, and barriers to prevent movement freely throughout a building, department, or area. Seclusion is a further escalation of environmental restraint to where the person is isolated or restrained into an environment that also prevents free movement.

A frequently cited guideline, the NICE Guidelines, from the NHS of England is an extensive advisory publication to assist with staff training and implementation of both chemical and mechanical restraints in ABDs in the setting of mental health problems [23]. This guideline may also be relevant to those who do not have diagnosed mental health pathology [23]. The guidelines are targeted "for adults older than 18, children younger than 12, and ages 13-17 with a mental health problem who are currently within mental health, health, and community settings".

It is important to utilize pre-initiation measurements to mitigate or reduce occurrence of agitation. The implementation of chemical restraint (rapid tranquillization), physical restraints, and seclusion should only be considered after de-escalation strategies are attempted and are unsuccessful [31]. There is no strong evidence concerning the efficacy of these three interventions in ABDs, but the following description of restraint application and monitoring is formulated in the setting of best available data [31]. De-escalation techniques should also be continually employed during this process as they are used in conjunction with other interventions. Continual use of de-escalation techniques throughout the process of restraint will help facilitate restraint placement and minimize agitation [23, 31].

Chemical restraints can be administered intramuscularly (IM) or intravenously (IV) when oral medication is unavailable or not a feasible option when the patient's agitation needs to be treated rapidly. In accordance with the algorithms noted in the NICE Guidelines, some of the most commonly used therapies for ABD is IM Lorazepam alone or the combination of IM haloperidol and promethazine [23]. However, the available options and combinations are numerous and ever growing. Broadly, the available chemical restraints can be categorized into first-generation antipsychotics, second-generation antipsychotics, benzodiazepines, and other [7].

The first-generation antipsychotics (typical) block dopamine receptors in the central nervous system. This class of medication can be further divided into high and low potency agents [7]. The high potency agents include: fluphenazine, haloperidol, loxapine, perphenazine, pimozide, thiothixene and trifluoperazine [7]. The low potency agents consist of chlorpromazine and thioridazine. These medications are effective but carry the risk of extrapyramidal syndromes (EPS) more commonly noted in the high-potency agents [7].

The second-generation antipsychotics (atypical) partially block dopamine and serotonin receptors. These medications, in comparison to first generation agents, have decreased rates of EPS, hyperprolactinemia, and movement disorders [7]. Despite this improved side effective profile, these medications are not without limitations. Prolonged use of these medication are associated with hyperglycemia and dyslipidemia as well as increased risk of cardiovascular disease [7]. The common agents within this group of medications are risperidone, olanzapine, quetiapine, ziprasidone, and aripiprazole.

The benzodiazepines are another class of medications that possess rapid anxiolytic and sedative properties. They also possess potential side effects of respiratory depression, hyper-salvia, and ataxia [7]. The most commonly used benzodiazepines are lorazepam, diazepam and midazolam.

Several other medications have been found to be effective in inducing sedation. Promethazine, an antihistamine, has been shown to be effective when utilized in combination with haloperidol. The combination of haloperidol-promethazine is the recommended first line medications of for rapid tranquilization in ABDs if no contraindications are present [23]. The purported mechanism of action for this drug mixture is to speed both the sedative and antimuscarinic effects of promethazine [7].

Although these various medication categories are commonly used in the ED for chemical restraint, providers must account for the patient's past medical history, possible intoxication, and interaction with other medications as well as total dose of daily medications. For example, Haloperidol-Promethazine or other QT prolonging medications should not be given to patients with prolonged QT intervals on ECG [7]. Medications should also be ordered as single doses as opposed to PRN to avoid inadvertent administrations and to ensure that appropriate response to medications is obtained.

If chemical restraint measures fail, care may be escalated to the use of physical restraints. Physical restraints are the next and often final option employed by available staff. Physical restraint can refer to two main categories: manual restraints in which the patient's body is held by other people or the utilization of devices and appliances. Both types of physical restraints are meant to assist the patient by preventing bodily harm to themselves or others.

The initiation of physical restraints can be conducted in a variety of manners. Traditionally, the camisole or straight jacket was used as a primary physical restraint [7]. Another option is to fasten the patient to a chair often referred to as ambulatory restraint [7]. However, 4- and 5-point restraints are most frequently used in the modern ED and will be the focus of this chapter's discussion of physical restraint. The four "points" of this restraint methods refer to the immobilization of both hands and both feet. 5-point restraint includes the previously mentioned four points with the addition of the chest. The mobility limiting agents are often leather and cloth straps with soft padding where they meet the skin to minimize the occurrence of skin breakdown or trauma. A principle of "only as necessary" should be employed with regards to restraint use and the patient's limitation should be as low as possible until the need for restraint is no longer needed. A host of factors should be considered in the sequence of applying restraints and continuous monitoring is imperative.

As with all procedures in the ED, proper management of the airway, breathing, and circulation is paramount during the application of physical restraints. The team leader should remain at the head of the bed while providing support and stabilization to the head and neck when appropriate [31]. This team member should direct the group in order that airway and breathing compromise can be evaluated and/or prevented during the process of restraint application. Vital signs should be continually monitored during this process to assess for acute decompensation or need for further medical intervention during the application of restraints.

The team leader is required to provide support and stabilization to the head as restraint application can have high morbidity and mortality including the potential for positional asphyxia [32]. Reduction in breathing is noted to occur less often when the patient was in supine positioning compared to prone [32]. The team leader should make sure to convey to the team that the patient should remain in the supine position during application of physical restraints [32]. Special consideration should be given to patients with pre-existing medical conditions (namely cardiac and respiratory disease) or also have been prescribed high-dose antipsychotics [32].

If restraints are being applied, one should employ an "all-or-none" philosophy to the restraint devices. Regarding either 4- or 5-point restraints, the team should apply all restraints to the patient. The freedom of one or multiple limbs can present a situation in which the patient can harm themselves, harm the staff, or damage the environment in which they are receiving care. To limit kicking and thrashing while in restraints, staff can employ a cross anchoring pattern with respect to the lower extremities. Staff can fasten the right leg to the left corner of the bed and the left leg to the right corner of the bed. Note that the patient should be maintained in the supine position during this fastening for minimization of risks discussed above. The devices for restraint should be attached to areas of the bed that move freely with bed repositioning (namely elevation of the head of the bed) [33].

During the process of restraint application, it is imperative to remember that the team is still providing care to an individual. Healthcare providers should make reasonable attempts to maintain patient privacy and mitigate humiliating factors. These factors should be considered when the intervention is occurring, and maintenance of dignity and privacy should be accommodated when possible. The level of applied force should be appropriate and proportional to the situation unfolding before health care professionals. Force should only be applied for the minimum amount of time that it is required. Although the situations are often fluid and rapidly evolving, care should be taken to minimize painful techniques. Although pain has no therapeutic role, it may be used when immediate danger or harm to health care professionals and staff is present. It is never the goal to enact a painful stimulus to a patient, however under certain circumstances it may be necessary for the defense and preservation of ED individual safety.

Following the conclusion of restraints, it is important for the team to be lead in a post-incident debrief and review of the ABD. The debrief provides an opportunity to review the factors leading up to the event, the performance of the team during the event, and areas for improvement. This debrief provides a forum to identify and evaluate potential risks, to address physical harms to staff, and evaluate the emotional impact to staff and bystanders. This debrief allows bystanders to discuss and process the events that occurred. It also gives active members an opportunity to discuss with non-active staff. Debrief engenders an area of safety, relaxation, and a return to previous activities and tasks [7, 31].

5. Restraint maintenance

After the decision to initiate patient restraint, the choice of restrain has been agreed upon, and the patient has been adequately secured, documentation and reassessments are the hallmark components of physical restrain maintenance. Restraint documentation frequency has been cited with intervals ranging from 15 minutes to hourly [5, 7, 31, 33–36]. These time frames are constructed with the intention of prompting frequent reassessments with the desired goal of termination of restraint utilization as soon as possible.

It is paramount that after administration of restraints (both chemical or physical), the patient's vital signs, hydration, and mental status are documented. Documentation should also include the need for continued restraint utilization, failed alternatives that resulted in the initiation of physical restraint, number of limbs restrained, the type of restraint utilized, the time of application, the mental status of the patient (orientation, fear, anger, and aggression before, during, and after restraint), the patient's response to restraint, and the presence/occurrence of any injuries during or after restraint [33]. The patient should also be continually observed if they appear asleep/sedated, have other illicit substance onboard, have a concerning past medical history, or have experienced harm because of the intervention [33].

For patients that are chemically restrained, care should be taken to reassess the patient after each dose of medication. PRN orders should be avoided to prevent oversedation and cumulative effects of medication administration as mentioned in the previous sections. PRN ordering schemes can potentially limit the ability of providers to assess levels of agitation correctly while potentially masking other complications hidden under the guise of sedation.

For those patients that are physically restrained, care should be taken to the areas of restraint fastening. These devices should be unlocked and unfastened one at a time in a sequential order to evaluate for skin break down or extremity trauma secondary to the restraint application. The patient should be able to move and range the extremity every two hours [33]. A detailed examination and evaluation of neurovascular status of this extremity should be performed in conjunction with this extremity assessment while restraints are in place [7, 33].

Physical examination of the patient during reassessment should focus on core areas that include but are not limited to the following systems: respiratory, cardiovascular, integumentary, and nervous. Respiratory evaluation should include comments on respiratory rate, work of breathing, airway patency, and respiratory rhythm. Cardiovascular evaluation should document heart rate and rhythm, presence and palpation of distal pulses, and capillary refill. Integumentary evaluation should comment on skin color, temperature, presence of wounds, or presence of edema. Nervous system documentation should portray the patient's orientation and level of consciousness, mobility, sensation, and presence of nervous deficits.

The patients position and location within the restraints should also be re-assessed during evaluation. The patient's bed should remain at the lowest height and remain locked in position [33]. The size of the restraint device should be proportional to the patients habitus and the patient should be placed in a position that minimizes the occurrence of neurovascular insult. Fasteners should be rechecked to make sure they are appropriately connected and that knots can be rapidly discontinued in emergent situations [33].

Patients should be closely monitored with a preference for direct observation. The presence of a direct observation (sometimes colloquially called "one-to-one") enables continuous assessment of the need for restraint or resolution of an ABD.

6. Restraint discontinuation and resource de-escalation

With continual monitoring and reassessment of patients, the overarching goal is to have the patient removed from restraints as soon as it is safe for the patient and staff to do so [37]. It is recognized that the utilization of a direct observer while the patient's restrained and the repeated, frequent need for reassessment and documentation can be onerous and deplete ED resources. For these and other reasons, it is advantageous to discontinue restraint orders as soon as possible.

7. Conclusion

This chapter addressed the epidemiological factors associated with increasing aggression and behavioral violence noted in the health care system. Due to the increasing prevalence of ABDs that put patients and providers at risk, this chapter reviewed both preventative strategies and interventions to minimize patient and staff harm,

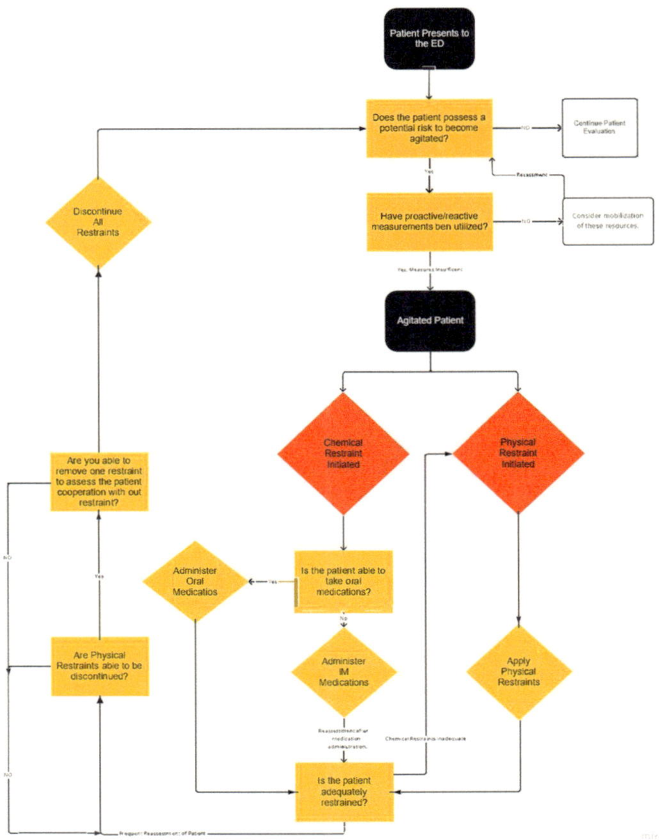

Figure 1.
Proposed workflow algorithm for the management of the acutely agitated patient in the ED. This figure acts as a visual aid to illustrate a flow of thinking and management questions that should be asked and answered throughout the evaluation of an agitated patient. Please reference the "Initiation of Restraints" Section for options on IM and IV Medications during utilization of this flowchart. Flowchart was created with the utilization of MIRO.com software (http://www.miro.com Last accessed on 12, August 2022).

reviewed the factors and considerations entailed in the application of restraints, and discussed the importance of reassessment and eventual restraint discontinuation. The provided flowchart (**Figure 1**) provides a condensed version of the logical progression a provider should consider in ABDs. As discussed throughout this chapter, the best strategy is to prevent ABD. However, there are tools and approaches that providers can utilize in the best interest of the patient to maintain the safety of the patient and health care providers during the management and care of a patient with ABD.

Acknowledgements

Figure construction was possible through the utilization of MIRO online software.

Conflicts of interest

The authors declare no conflicts of interest.

Author details

Abby White and Christopher Kustera*
Saint Luke's University Health Network, Easton, United States of America

*Address all correspondence to: christopher.kustera@sluhn.org

References

[1] Cui N, Qiu R, Zhang Y, Chen D, Zhang H, Rao H, et al. Why are physical restraints still in use? A qualitative descriptive study from Chinese critical care clinicians' perspectives. BMJ Open. 2021;**11**(11):e055073

[2] Weiland T, Ivory S, Hutton J. Managing acute Behavioural disturbances in the emergency department using the environment, policies and practices: A systematic review. The Western Journal of Emergency Medicine. 2017;**18**(4):647-661

[3] Ye J, Wang C, Xiao A, Xia Z, Yu L, Lin J, et al. Physical restraint in mental health nursing: A concept analysis. International Journal of Nursing Sciences. 2019;**6**(3):343-348

[4] Chieze M, Hurst S, Kaiser S, Sentissi O. Effects of seclusion and restraint in adult psychiatry: A systematic review. Frontiers in Psychiatry. 2019;**10**:491

[5] Eltaliawi AG, El-Shinawi M, Comer A, Hamazah S, Hirshon JM. Restraint use among selected hospitalized elderly patients in Cairo, Egypt. BMC Research Notes. 2017;**10**(1):633

[6] Gunawardena S. The attitudes towards the use of restraint and restrictive intervention amongst healthcare staff on acute medical and frailty wards—A brief literature review. Geriatrics. 2019;**4**(3):50

[7] Ziaei M, Massoudifar A, Rajabpour-Sanati A, Pourbagher-Shahri AM, Abdolrazaghnejad A. Management of violence and aggression in emergency environment; a narrative review of 200 related articles. Advanced Journal of Emergency Medicine. 2018;**3**(1):e7. [Internet]. [cited 2022 Jul 16]; (In press). DOI: 10.22114/ajem.v0i0.117

[8] Wong AH, Sabounchi NS, Roncallo HR, Ray JM, Heckmann R. A qualitative system dynamics model for effects of workplace violence and clinician burnout on agitation management in the emergency department. BMC Health Services Research. 2022;**22**(1):75

[9] Roennfeldt H, Wyder M, Byrne L, Hill N, Randall R, Hamilton B. Subjective experiences of mental health crisis Care in Emergency Departments: A narrative review of the qualitative literature. International Journal of Environmental Research and Public Health. 2021;**18**(18):9650

[10] Robins LM, Lee DCA, Bell JS, Srikanth V, Möhler R, Hill KD, et al. Definition and measurement of physical and chemical restraint in long-term care: A systematic review. International Journal of Environmental Research and Public Health. 2021;**18**(7):3639

[11] Richardson SK, Ardagh MW, Morrison R, Grainger PC. Management of the aggressive emergency department patient: Non-pharmacological perspectives and evidence base. Open Access Emergency Medicine. 2019;**11**:271-290

[12] Ramacciati N, Ceccagnoli A, Addey B, Lumini E, Rasero L. Violence towards emergency nurses: A narrative review of theories and frameworks. International Emergency Nursing. 2018;**39**:2-12

[13] Chou HJ, Tseng KY. The experience of emergency nurses caring for patients with mental illness: A qualitative study. International Journal of Environmental Research and Public Health. 2020;**17**(22):8540

[14] Wong AH, Ray JM, Rosenberg A, Crispino L, Parker J, McVaney C, et al. Experiences of individuals who were physically restrained in the emergency department. JAMA Network Open. 2020;**3**(1):e1919381

[15] Bessey LJ, Radue RM, Chapman EN, Boyle LL, Shah MN. Behavioral health needs of older adults in the emergency department. Clinics in Geriatric Medicine. 2018;**34**(3):469-489

[16] Manuel MM, Feng S, Yen K, Patel F. The agitated pediatric patient located in the emergency department: The APPLIED observational study. Journal of the American College of Emergency Physicians Open. 2022;**3**(3):e12766. [Internet] [cited 2022 Jul 16]. Available from: https://onlinelibrary.wiley.com/doi/10.1002/emp2.12766

[17] Peltzer-Jones J, Nordstrom K, Currier G, Berlin J, Singh C, Schneider S. A research agenda for assessment and Management of Psychosis in emergency department patients. The Western Journal of Emergency Medicine. 2019;**20**(2):403-408

[18] Kersting XAK, Hirsch S, Steinert T. Physical harm and death in the context of coercive measures in psychiatric patients: A systematic review. Frontiers in Psychiatry. 2019;**10**:400

[19] Celofiga A, Kores Plesnicar B, Koprivsek J, Moskon M, Benkovic D, Gregoric KH. Effectiveness of De-escalation in reducing aggression and coercion in acute psychiatric units. A cluster randomized study. Front Psychiatry. 2022;**13**:856153

[20] Wong AH, Whitfill T, Ohuabunwa EC, Ray JM, Dziura JD, Bernstein SL, et al. Association of race/ethnicity and other demographic characteristics with use of physical restraints in the emergency department. JAMA Network Open. 2021;**4**(1):e2035241

[21] Siegrist-Dreier S, Barbezat I, Thomann S, Richter D, Hahn S, Schmitt K. Restraining patients in acute care hospitals—A qualitative study on the experiences of healthcare staff. Nursing Open. 2022;**9**(2):1311-1321

[22] Raveesh B, Gowda G, Gowda M. Alternatives to use of restraint: A path toward humanistic care. Indian Journal of Psychiatry. 2019;**61**(10):693

[23] National Institute for Health and Care Excellence. Violence and Aggression Short-Term Management in Mental Health, Health and Community Settings (Updated edition). NICE guideline NG10. 2015. [Internet]. [cited 2022 Aug 8]. Available from: https://www.nice.org.uk/guidance/ng10/evidence/full-guideline-pdf-70830253

[24] Morrison J, Hasselblad M, Kleinpell R, Buie R, Ariosto D, Hardiman E, et al. The disruptive bEhavior manageMEnt ANd prevention in hospitalized patients using a behaviORal intervention team (DEMEANOR) study protocol: A pragmatic, cluster, crossover trial for the Vanderbilt learning healthcare system investigators, Vanderbilt University. Trials. 2020;**21**(1):417

[25] Roppolo LP, Morris DW, Khan F, Downs R, Metzger J, Carder T, et al. Improving the management of acutely agitated patients in the emergency department through implementation of project BETA (best practices in the evaluation and treatment of agitation). Journal of the American College of Emergency Physicians Open. 2020;**1**(5):898-907

[26] Wong AH, Ray JM, Auerbach MA, Venkatesh AK, McVaney C, Burness D,

et al. Study protocol for the ACT response pilot intervention: Development, implementation and evaluation of a systems-based agitation code team (ACT) in the emergency department. BMJ Open. 2020;**10**(6):e036982

[27] Agboola IK, Coupet E, Wong AH. "The coats that we can take off and the ones we Can't": The role of trauma-informed care on race and bias during agitation in the emergency department. Annals of Emergency Medicine. 2021;**77**(5):493-498

[28] Berg SH, Rørtveit K, Walby FA, Aase K. Safe clinical practice for patients hospitalised in mental health wards during a suicidal crisis: Qualitative study of patient experiences. BMJ Open. 2020;**10**(11):e040088

[29] Hart KL, Pellegrini AM, Forester BP, Berretta S, Murphy SN, Perlis RH, et al. Distribution of agitation and related symptoms among hospitalized patients using a scalable natural language processing method. General Hospital Psychiatry. 2021;**68**:46-51

[30] Barnett S, Factors B. Associated with the use of seclusion in an inpatient psychiatric unit in Lilongwe, Malawi. Malawi Medical Journal. 2018;**30**(3):197

[31] Nelstrop L, Chandler-Oatts J, Bingley W, Bleetman T, Corr F, Cronin-Davis J, et al. A systematic review of the safety and effectiveness of restraint and seclusion as interventions for the short-term Management of Violence in adult psychiatric inpatient settings and emergency departments. Worldviews on Evidence-Based Nursing. 2006;**3**(1):8-18

[32] Walker H, Tulloch L. A "necessary evil": Staff perspectives of soft restraint kit use in a high-security hospital. Frontiers in Psychiatry. 2020;**11**:357

[33] SharifiA,ArsalaniN,Fallahi-KhoshknabM, Mohammadi-Shahbolaghi F. The principles of physical restraint use for hospitalized elderly people: An integrated literature review. Systematic Reviews. 2021;**10**(1):129

[34] Palese A, Longhini J, Businarolo A, Piccin T, Pitacco G, Bicego L. Between restrictive and supportive devices in the context of physical restraints: Findings from a large mixed-method study design. International Journal of Environmental Research and Public Health. 2021;**18**(23):12764

[35] Mulkey MA, Munro CL. Calming the agitated patient: Providing strategies to support clinicians. Medsurg Nursing Official Journal of Academic Medicine-Surgery Nurses. 2021;**30**(1):9-13

[36] de Bruijn W, Daams JG, van Hunnik FJG, Arends AJ, Boelens AM, Bosnak EM, et al. Physical and pharmacological restraints in hospital care: Protocol for a systematic review. Frontiers in Psychiatry. 2020;**10**:921

[37] American College of Emergency Physicians (ACEP). Use of patient restraints. Policy statement. Annals of Emergency Medicine. Nov 2014;**64**(5):574. DOI: 10.1016/j. annemergmed.2014.08.039. Epub 2014 Oct 22. PMID: 25669717

Chapter 6

Improving the Safety of Admitted Patients with Alcohol Use Disorder and Withdrawal

Clayton Korson and Thomas Nappe

Abstract

The aim of this chapter is to review the pathophysiology of alcohol withdrawal syndrome (AWS), discuss diagnostic strategies, identify clinical manifestations, outline appropriate management options, and address key patient safety considerations specifically as it applies to the hospitalized patient. Ethanol use causes substantial morbidity and mortality and is among the most widely abused substances in the world. Up to 40% of all hospitalized patients are at risk for suffering from alcohol withdrawal syndrome (AWS). AWS is a hyperdynamic syndrome with symptoms that can include anxiety, insomnia, tachycardia, hypertension, tremor, nausea, vomiting, seizures, coma, disability, and death. Several screening tools can help identify patients with alcohol use disorder and those at risk for AWS. Symptom based scoring systems, such as the Clinical Institute Withdrawal Assessment for Alcohol (CIWA) or Severity of Ethanol Withdrawal Score (SEWS) score, are also available for guiding treatment. Treatment options should primarily consist of Gamma-Aminobutyric Acid (GABA) agonists, including benzodiazepines and barbiturate (mainly phenobarbital) medications, however other adjunctive therapies are also available. The most important patient safety principles for the hospitalized patient with AWS include early assessment, identification, and intervention, treatment of associated medical and psychiatric complications, as well as a comprehensive multi-disciplinary approach.

Keywords: Alcohol withdrawal syndrome, patient safety, phenobarbital, toxicology, addiction medicine

1. Introduction

Ethanol is the one of the most widely abused substances in the world and is associated with substantial morbidity and mortality. Approximately 85% of adults over the age of 18 report alcohol consumption in the United States, and annually ~90,000 people die from alcohol related causes [1]. Nearly 15 million Americans meet criteria for alcohol use disorder (AUD), and it is estimated that up to 40% of hospitalized patients suffer from AUD, putting them at risk for alcohol withdrawal syndrome (AWS) and other related conditions [2]. AWS is a spectrum illness that ranges from early or mild symptoms (anxiety, headache, nausea, sleep disturbances) to later, severe, life threatening complications including seizures, dysautonomia, coma, and death [2]. It is critical for healthcare professionals to be able to recognize and understand key principles related to AWS, as well as the health conditions and complications associated with alcohol use disorder, in order to collaboratively ensure the safety and wellness of the hospitalized patient.

2. Methodology

A comprehensive literature search was used to obtain evidence to support this manuscript. Sources included internet-based search engines such as PubMed, Google™ Scholar, and SCOPUS™ in addition to other medical textbooks, commercialized medical resources (EMRAP™, UpToDate™, EMCRIT™), and internationally recognized societal guidelines (*American Society of Addiction Medicine, American College of Emergency Physicians, American College of Medical Toxicology*). Common search terms included but were not limited to "alcohol withdrawal syndrome," "complicated alcohol withdrawal syndrome," "inpatient management of alcohol withdrawal syndrome," "pathophysiology of alcohol withdrawal," "alcohol withdrawal seizures," "delirium tremens," "phenobarbital and alcohol withdrawal syndrome," "CIWA," "SEWS," Wernicke's Encephalopathy," "medical management of alcohol withdrawal syndrome," alcohol withdrawal syndrome complications," "patient safety and alcohol withdrawal." Our search initially queried more than one million sources; sources were screened and appraised based on their quality of evidence and relevancy to alcohol withdrawal syndrome in the hospitalized patient. This narrowed down the literature search to approximately 100 articles which were further consolidated based on redundancy, resulting in the 33 sources included in the chapter.

3. Pathophysiology

Ethanol (C_2H_5OH) is a two-carbon molecule with an attached hydroxyl group. Various alcoholic beverages contain between 5 and 40% of ethanol by concentration; one standard drink in the United States is defined as 14 grams of ethanol [3]. The molecule is slightly lipophilic and can penetrate the blood brain barrier as a result. The Central Nervous System (CNS) functions via a delicate balancing act between inhibitory γ-aminobutyric acid (GABA) receptors and excitatory glutamic N-methyl-D-aspartate (NMDA) receptors. Ethanol acts as a CNS depressant by primarily augmenting GABA receptors and antagonizing excitatory NMDA receptors [4]. At low CNS concentrations ethanol induces behavioral excitation and euphoria, whereas at higher concentrations, ataxia, drowsiness, and slurred speech are common. Longstanding alcohol consumption causes physical tolerance (increasing doses to achieve the same effect) in a multitude of CNS receptor sites, including NMDA, GABA, serotonin (5HT), glycine, G-protein coupled rectifying potassium channels, as well as several others [5]. Ethanol also directly binds to glutamate, thereby enhancing its inhibitory effect on the brain [6]. Several studies have demonstrated that specifically the δ-$GABA_A$ receptors appear to be most sensitive to ethanol [5]. These are most highly concentrated in the cerebellum, cortex, thalamic nuclei and brain stem, which correlates with the clinical manifestations of ethanol intoxication. Prolonged ethanol exposure also results in specific adaptive changes to GABA receptor concentration and subunit composition. As an example, decreased α1 and γ2 GABA subunit expression, as seen in those with AUD, is theorized to directly affect CNS inhibitory tone [5]. Additionally, there is an upregulation of excitatory NMDA receptors. As a result, chronically consuming ethanol can predispose individuals to a baseline excitatory state [5]. Ultimately this disruption of homeostasis serves as the basis for AWS.

When a chronic ethanol stimulus is abruptly discontinued, the underlying molecular changes yield AWS. CNS excitatory activity becomes relatively unopposed. Dysautonomia results from an enhanced sympathetic nervous system activity and manifests as tachycardia, hypertension, hyperthermia, tremor, nausea, and vomiting [7]. Alcohol withdrawal related seizures are theorized to originate primarily from excitatory activity in the brainstem (specifically the inferior colliculus), although evidence also supports involvement of the hippocampus [5]. Additionally, repeated episodes of withdrawal may result in permanent epileptic changes in the brain, thus lowering the seizure threshold and putting individuals at even higher risk of AWS induced seizures [5]. Dopamine signaling, another neurotransmitter implicated in AWS, is increased as well, and appears to be responsible for the symptoms of alcoholic hallucinosis [6]. "Kindling" is another phenomenon associated with AWS, where neurons becoming increasingly sensitive, and as a result, subsequent episodes of AWS can be more severe [5, 7]. Outside of its CNS manifestations, AWS and alcohol use disorder more broadly is also associated with varying degrees of electrolyte abnormalities, metabolic derangements, nutritional deficiencies, coagulopathies and many other co-morbidities due to the toxic effects of longstanding ethanol ingestion as will be detailed in subsequent sections.

In summary, neuro-adaptive changes resulting from longstanding, regular ethanol use predispose to an excitatory neurological state, that cascades through the spectrum of AWS following cessation of ethanol. As a result, patients suffer from a range of neurologic symptoms, some of which can be life threatening. It is critical that clinicians are familiar with these manifestations and can diagnose and treat them rapidly.

4. Diagnostics

AUD is a medical condition where one experiences difficulty in stopping or controlling the use of alcohol, despite experiencing adverse social, occupational, or health consequences [8].

AUD is a significant patient safety issue in the hospitalized patient, associated with morbidity and mortality, especially when it goes undiagnosed or undertreated. Although many patients present self-reporting alcohol use disorder or withdrawal while requesting treatment, many present for new or related illnesses and complications without proper disclosure, risk stratification, assessment, or treatment and either progress to alcohol withdrawal or have other conditions that mask it due to overlapping symptomatology. For example, a patient may present with pancreatitis and not fully inform of recent or regular alcohol use. Others may present later in the disease course with symptoms or complications that may cause the clinician to overlook AUD as an etiology. Another example would be a new onset seizure in an encephalopathic patient, prompting a neurological evaluation and empiric treatment with ineffective antiepileptic agents, leaving the alcohol withdrawal untreated. A patient who fell and suffered a subdural hematoma may not be suspected of recent intoxication or alcohol related neuropathy as the cause of the fall and can then be at risk for experiencing alcohol withdrawal. These patients will be at risk of developing severe alcohol withdrawal that can result in severe complications, including permanent disability and death.

Clinicians should inquire about a patient's drinking habits, including quantity and duration of alcohol consumption, and any history of AWS to identify patients with AUD and to gauge the likelihood of AWS. Several questionnaires are useful in aiding this history taking [9]. Once screening has been performed, clinicians can then utilize additional scoring tools for risk stratification and therapy. The various screening tools that can be used for identifying alcohol use disorder in the hospital include AUDIT (Alcohol Use Disorders Identification Test), AUDIT-C (the Shortened Alcohol Use Disorders Identification Test), the CAGE questionnaire (Cut down Annoyed, Guilty, Eye-opener), the TACE (Tolerance, Annoyed Cut down, Eye-opener; mainly for pregnant patients) and SBIRT (Screening and Brief Intervention Tool). Although the in-depth description of these screening tools is beyond the focus of this chapter, it is important that hospital systems utilize a screening tool to assist in identifying and diagnosing patients with alcohol use disorder, so that they can then risk stratify who may be at risk for withdrawal and implement a treatment plan, all while evaluating and treating for common comorbidities. Risk stratification can also be performed utilizing the PAWSS score (The Prediction of Alcohol Withdrawal Severity Scale) while the most common treatment assessment tool is Clinical Institute Withdrawal Assessment (CIWA). These tools are further described in subsequent sections.

Comorbidities and other clinical clues useful for identifying alcohol use disorder may include common diagnostic findings, such as transaminitis (AST > ALT in 2–3:1 ratio, generally <500 U/L), macrocytic anemia, thrombocytopenia, and electrolyte derangements – most commonly hyponatremia, hypokalemia, and hypocalcemia; and therefore, QT prolongation and risk of dysrhythmia. Commonly associated conditions include traumatic injuries, pancreatitis, gastritis, gastrointestinal bleeding, alcoholic ketoacidosis, malnutrition, dehydration, acute kidney injury, hypertension. All of these findings should be reason to consider a patient for potentially having alcohol use disorder and being at risk for withdrawal.

Evaluation of the patient identified with alcohol use disorder or withdrawal syndrome should include electrocardiogram, complete blood count, complete metabolic panel, magnesium (especially if hypokalemic), INR, lipase if any gastrointestinal symptoms, serum ethanol concentration, and if any alteration of mental status, computed tomography of brain. CT imaging of brain should be considered particularly if any concern for traumatic injury. Further evaluation for cardiac ischemia or cardiomyopathy should also be considered. Obtaining a serum ethanol concentration is important as is it not possible for clinicians to commonly predict degree of intoxication based on assessment of clinical sobriety. An elevated serum ethanol concentration in a presenting patient should be reason to evaluate for alcohol use disorder, and should prompt concern for possible withdrawal. Although patients may begin to withdraw at elevated serum ethanol concentrations, many may not start to withdraw for easily six hours after they metabolize all their ethanol. In this case, a predictive timeline can be generated, utilizing the average ethanol metabolism of 15 mg/kg/hr., to determine how long to observe for symptomatology.

The PAWSS score is a clinical scoring tool that can be utilized to assess patients identified with AUD to risk stratify the likelihood of developing AWS (**Table 1**). Severity can then be monitored with CIWA or SEWS [10, 11]. A PAWSS score < 4 portends a low risk of moderate to severe AWS, whereas a score > 4 places a patient at high risk of experiencing severe AWS [10]. The prospective validation study of PAWSS resulted in a sensitivity of 93% and specificity of 99.5% in predicting severe withdrawal for hospitalized patients, making it a highly useful tool for the modern-day practitioner in treating AWS [12].

	Yes	No
Has the patient been intoxicated or drunk in the past 30 days?		
Has the patient EVER undergone alcohol use disorder rehabilitation treatment or treatment for alcoholism? (Inpatient or outpatient settings)		
Has the patient EVER experienced ANY previous episodes of alcohol withdrawal?		
Has the patient EVER experienced blackouts from drinking?		
Has the patient EVER experienced alcohol withdrawal seizures?		
Has the patient EVER experienced delirium tremens?		
Has the patient combined alcohol with other "downers" in the past 90 days?		
Has the patient combined alcohol with ANY other substance of abuse in the past 90 days?		
Was the patient's blood alcohol level ≥ 200 (mg/dL) on presentation?		
Is there evidence of increased autonomic activity? (Increased heart rate > 120, hypertension tremors, agitation, etc..)		

Source: [10].
Each "Yes" answered confers +1 point.

Table 1.
Prediction of Alcohol Withdrawal severity scale (PAWSS).

Question	Score Range
"Do you feel sick to your stomach? Have you vomited?"	0 to 7
Paroxysmal sweats	0 to 7
Agitation	0 to 7
"Does your head feel different? Does it feel like there's a band around your head?"	0 to 7
"Do you feel nervous?"	0 to 7
Tremor	0 to 7
"Does the light appear to be too bright? Is its color different? Does it hurt your eyes? Are you seeing anything that is disturbing to you? Are you seeing things you know are not there?"	0 to 7
"Have you any itching, pins and needles sensations, any burning, any numbness, or do you feel bugs crawling on or under your skin?"	0 to 7
"Are you more aware of sounds around you? Are they harsh? Do they frighten you? Are you hearing anything that is disturbing to you? Are you hearing things you know are not there?"	0 to 7
"What day is today? What is this place?"	0 to 4

Source: [13].
Range of 0 to 67 with higher scores indicating higher severity of AWS.

Table 2.
Clinical Institute of Alcohol Withdrawal Score – Revised (CIWA-R).

Once a patient is identified as potentially having AUD and is then risk stratified for possibly developing AWS, several scoring systems are available for further monitoring and treatment. The revised Clinical Institute Withdrawal Assessment for Alcohol Scale

(CIWA) was among the first scores designed to appropriately guide treatment for AWS [13]. The CIWA score has been adopted across numerous health systems worldwide and is the most common clinical tool utilized for AWS. The score takes several minutes to calculate and ranges from 0 to 67 with severity of withdrawal being associated with higher scores (scores >20 indicates severe AWS). The questionnaire assesses for nausea, diaphoresis, tremor, hallucinations, among other symptoms indicative of AWS (**Table 2**). The score can then be tied to escalating doses of medications, such as benzodiazepines, for symptom triggered treatment. CIWA has been shown to result in more reliable benzodiazepine (BZD) dosing, decreased length of hospital stay, and decreased rate of severe complications when compared to unscored symptom-based dosing [14]. However, there are limitations to CIWA as several components of the questionnaire are subjective in nature and may result in variability between clinicians.

The Severity of Ethanol Withdrawal Scale (SEWS) is another clinical scoring tool that can be used to guide treatment for AWS [15]. Similar to CIWA, SEWS generates a calculated score ranging from 0 to 24 with higher scores (scores >13) indicating severe AWS (**Table 3**). SEWS is not as often utilized as CIWA currently, however in a 2019 quality assurance study, it was shown to decrease hospital length of stay by one day by allowing for more aggressive BZD treatment without over sedation risk when compared to CIWA [15]. SEWS also showed to be more objective, utilizing vital signs, and more easily performed by provider, likely since it has less questions. Further prospective studies are needed for external validation, however in the meantime, initial results appear promising in using SEWS to guide treatment for AWS.

To summarize, the three clinical scoring tools presented (CIWA, SEWS, PAWSS) are crucial when it comes to risk stratifying and treating AWS. In addition, clinicians must be mindful of the many co-morbidities that patient's suffering from AWS frequently present with and obtain appropriate diagnostic testing for these as well. Appropriately recognizing AUD, AWS and related co-morbidities is paramount for patient safety.

Question	Score if positive
Anxiety: Do you feel that something bad is about to happen to you right now?	0 or 3
NAUSEA and DRY HEAVES or VOMITING?	0 or 3
SWEATING (includes moist palms, sweating now)?	0 or 2
TREMOR: with arms extended, eyes closed	0 or 2
AGITATION: fidgety, restless, pacing	0 or 3
DISORIENTATION: Knows name and place, but not date Knows name only	0 or 1 0 or 3
HALLUCINATIONS: Auditory only (check for major psychiatric disorder) Visual, tactile, olfactory, gustatory (any)	0 or 1 0 or 3
VITAL SIGNS: ANY of the following: 1. Pulse >100 2) diastolic BP >90, 3) temp >37.6 C	0 or 3

Source: [15].
Range of 0 to 22 with higher scores indicating higher severity of AWS.

Table 3.
Severity of ethanol Withdrawal scale (SEWS).

5. Alcohol withdrawal syndrome

AWS can be considered a spectral illness, ranging from early/mild to late/severe, with additional complications, including delirium tremens (DT) and possibly Wernicke's Encephalopathy (WE) and Wernicke-Korsakoff Syndrome (WKS) which are generally considered to be secondary to thiamine (vitamin B1) deficiency. WE is often reversible with prompt recognition and treatment but can progress to the less reversible WKS if inadequately treated. It is important to realize that for patients with mild AUD, symptoms may never progress beyond mild, while for patients with severe AUD, early withdrawal may start with severe symptoms and rapidly progress. Additionally, DT is an entirely avoidable phenomenon and results from either late presentation or suboptimal treatment.

5.1 Mild: moderate AWS

In classic AWS, patients typically become symptomatic 6-hours after their last drink (or if they have significantly decreased their ethanol intake) but can take up to 24-hours before they become apparent [16]. Symptoms may begin mildly or can abruptly start as more severe grades of AWS [17]. Nausea, vomiting, and diaphoresis are common, as well as tremors, headaches, anxiety, and insomnia. Autonomic dysfunction may develop as well, including hypertension, tachycardia, and hyperthermia. It is important to recognize that patient's taking certain medication classes, such as beta-blockers or alpha-2 agonists, may mask their autonomic dysfunction [17]. Tactile, auditory, and visual hallucinations may be present in up to 25% of AWS patient's, however patient's sensorium often remains intact (as opposed to in alcoholic hallucinosis or organic psychosis) [17]. Mild to moderate AWS usually dissipates between 2 and 7 days and often without treatment [17]. These patients may not even present to healthcare facilities for evaluation or treatment and it is likely an underdiagnosed phenomenon.

5.2 Moderate: severe AWS

Moderate-severe AWS includes many of the symptoms described in mild-moderate AWS; however, symptoms are severe and may be refractory to treatment. Classic symptom (tachycardia, hypertension, tremor, nausea, vomiting, diaphoresis, anxiety) are notably worse and will likely require more aggressive treatment regimens. Hallucinations may become persistent, progressing into alcoholic hallucinosis (AH). AH occurs in up to 8% of patients and typically 12- to 24-hours after a patient's last drink [18, 19]. Neuroleptic medication has been shown to worsen hallucinations in AH and should be avoided [19].

Wernicke's Encephalopathy, the triad of confusion, ophthalmoplegia, and cerebellar symptoms (such as ataxia), may also become apparent in moderate-severe AWS. Seizures can occur in up to 10% of patients with AWS [17]. AWS seizures generally occur 24- to 48- hours after alcohol cessation. Seizure activity includes generalized tonic-clonic jerks and can lack a post-ictal period [17, 18]. AWS seizures are notoriously difficult to treat with traditional antiepileptic agents and may portend a worse prognosis, including progression into delirium tremens, a form of agitated delirium, the most severe manifestation of AWS [17]. Often escalating doses of BZD and other adjunct therapy is needed in these cases, and intensive care management may be warranted.

5.3 Delirium tremens

Delirium Tremens (DT), a form of agitated delirium, is the most severe form of AWS and occurs in up to 5% of patients [19–21]. Symptoms generally occur in the 2–4-day time range from a patient's last known ingestion. DT as a syndrome includes severe, rapid changes in cognition, memory, consciousness, and perception in addition to extreme autonomic distress including malignant hypertension and hyperthermia [17, 20]. Hallucinations, disorientation, psychosis, and coma are hallmarks of DT. Symptoms are generally refractory to treatment, may last up to one week or longer, and may be lethal. The mortality rate for DT is between 1% and 5%, generally secondary to medical complications such as aspiration or myocardial infarction [17]. Treatment for DT requires the maximum therapeutic options available to treating clinicians. Aggressive BZD dosing (often defined as >20-40 mg diazepam or equivalent per hour for severe CIWA or SEWS), phenobarbital, and adjunct therapies such as dexmedetomidine, propofol, or ketamine may be necessary. Endotracheal intubation and intensive care management are sometimes needed for patients with DT. Ultimately, DT is the most severe form of AWS and causes substantial morbidity and mortality. From a patient safety perspective, it is important to realize that DT is not a routine outcome of the spectrum of alcohol withdrawal and can be completely prevented with early, adequate treatment of AWS [22].

6. Management

6.1 Disposition

Management of alcohol withdrawal occurs in a variety of settings, the most appropriate being a withdrawal management facility, or commonly known as a "detox center," or a hospital (note that "detox" refers to management of withdrawal symptoms, not actual detoxification, which is the removal of an agent). The authors do not generally recommend outpatient alcohol withdrawal management due to the difficulty in assessing mild versus early withdrawal with the risk of worsening, as well as difficulty with patient compliance. Patients may primarily seek withdrawal management and be appropriately placed in a detox facility that meets their level of medical needs or may occur in the hospital setting. Alcohol withdrawal often occurs in the hospital setting when patients present ill from their withdrawal symptoms and require admission, present for complications of alcohol use disorder (e.g., pancreatitis, trauma, etc.) and withdraw, or present for other medical problems requiring admission and have to suddenly discontinue consumption of alcohol. When alcohol use disorder or withdrawal are encountered in the hospital setting, a collaborative approach is recommended to assure patient safety and optimize patient care. This collaborative approach may include internal medicine, critical care, medical toxicology, addiction medicine, psychiatry, and case management.

Although the focus of this chapter is alcohol withdrawal in the hospital setting, it is important to realize there are withdrawal management facilities available to safely discontinue alcohol. The *American Society of Addiction Medicine* has designated four levels (1–4) of withdrawal management. Level 1 refers to ambulatory management with minimal on-site monitoring, and Level 4 corresponds to a medically managed inpatient therapy setting [16]. Generally, patients with a CIWA score < 10 may be managed in Level 1 settings, CIWA score of 10 to 18 in Level 2 or

Level 3 settings, and > 19 should be managed in a Level 4, resource rich environment [16]. Independent of a patient's symptoms, additional factors will influence the required treatment setting. Psychosocial factors, such as social support or suicide risk, may require a higher level of care. Additional considerations influencing the level of care include but are not limited to: co-substance dependence (opioids, tobacco, etc..), recent ethanol consumption, personal history of AWS or complicated withdrawal, and co-morbid illness such as cirrhosis, chronic obstructive pulmonary disease, congestive heart failure, epilepsy, or renal disease [16]. Patients who are older or pregnant are at higher risk of complications from AWS and benefit from more highly monitored settings [16]. Ultimately, this decision should be made on a case-by-case basis. If in question, it is always better to err on the side of caution and recommend a higher level of care.

Despite there being detox facilities available, many patients may still ultimately require withdrawal management in an inpatient hospital setting due to the aforementioned reasons. Additionally, patients with severe withdrawal, encephalopathy or additional complications may require intensive care. To assure patient safety, the authors recommend hospitals consider employing and collaborating with addiction specialists for consultation or primary management [16]. While withdrawal management facilities generally involve treatment from addiction specialists, opportunities commonly exist within hospitals to provide expert care from this specialty.

Once a treatment setting has been decided upon, general supportive care management should be followed concurrently with appropriate pharmacotherapy (as will be described in subsequent sections). Non-pharmacological options should be utilized, including a dark, quiet room with minimal stimulation [17]. Efforts should be made to frequently reassure patients. Psychiatric assessments for anxiety, insomnia, or suicidality should be conducted and treated appropriately. General supportive care often includes correction of electrolyte imbalances, hypoglycemia correction, hydration therapy (either oral or via fluid resuscitation), and thiamine and other B-vitamin supplementation. Typical thiamine dosing is 100 mg PO per day for 3 to 5 days and ideally should be given prior to, or in conjunction with, glucose supplementation to prevent precipitating (or worsening) Wernicke's Encephalopathy (this will be further elaborated upon in Section 5.3.3) [16, 17]. Patients should be monitored closely and informed regarding their treatment progress, including whether a higher-level treatment setting is indicated.

6.2 Treatment

6.2.1 Benzodiazepines (BZD): B

ZDs have long been considered the "gold standard" pharmacological treatment option for AWS. They act primarily by stimulating $GABA_A$ receptors by enhancing the *frequency* of chloride channel opening in the presence of GABA [16, 17]. BZDs have been shown to reduce the incidence of seizures, DT, and mortality in AWS [23]. BZDs may be delivered via intravenous, oral, or intramuscular routes, making it an advantageous drug in a variety of situations. Longer acting agents, such as diazepam or chlordiazepoxide, are preferred to allow for a theoretically smoother clinical course due to a proposed auto-tapering mechanism [16, 17]; however, they are all generally effective if dosed appropriately. Diazepam, when administered intravenously, has both the fastest onset and longest duration of action. Lorazepam, diazepam, and chlordiazepoxide are the most prescribed BZDs in treating AWS [16]. There is never a need to mix benzodiazepines and it can cloud the clinical picture and increase risk of rebound symptoms. Several different dosing strategies are available, including "fixed-dose", "loading-dose", and a "symptoms-triggered" strategies [17]. In fixed dosing, the chosen drug (e.g.10 mg Diazepam QID) is given regularly and then can be subsequently tapered by 25% on days 4 through 7 with liberal dosing as needed for breakthrough symptoms [17]. In a "symptom-triggered" plan (which is preferred), a chosen BZD (e.g. diazepam, lorazepam, chlordiazepoxide) is prescribed based on a patient's hourly CIWA or SEWS score, and doses are escalated as needed [24]. Tapering occurs through smaller doses as scoring decreases. Finally, in a "loading-dose" strategy, higher doses of a chosen BZD are administered until symptoms improve (e.g. Diazepam 20 mg, 40 mg, 60 mg, ...100 mg) to allow for a self-taper effect [25]. Regardless of strategy, when utilizing benzodiazepines, close monitoring is necessary to assure no recurrence of symptoms in the short term, and consideration of duration of action of chosen benzodiazepine should be considered in monitoring time. Prescribing BZDs in a symptom triggered fashion has been shown to reduce the total amount of BZD administered and shortens total therapy time, however no specific strategy is clearly superior [17, 24].

6.2.2 Barbiturates

Barbiturates, primarily phenobarbital, provide another valuable and safe option for effectively treating alcohol withdrawal. They act by stimulating $GABA_A$ but, unlike BZD, they increase *duration* of chloride channel opening and they do not require the presence of GABA [26]. Being able to directly stimulate the $GABA_A$ receptor without the presence of GABA may provide increased effectiveness over benzodiazepines in controlling symptoms [26]. Additionally, phenobarbital can decrease glutamate activity which thereby assists in treating the hyperdynamic state that results from upregulated NMDA receptor activity [27]. Phenobarbital also has a more predictable pharmacological profile, is more effective for preventing seizures than benzodiazepines, has less incidence of delirium, results in less progression of symptoms, decreases critical care utilization, [26, 28–31]. Phenobarbital does not need to be tapered as it is very long acting and self-tapers over the course of three to five days, thus generally outlasting the AWS disease process. There are various dosing regimens for phenobarbital. Initial doses of phenobarbital 10 mg/kg IV over thirty minutes may be utilized prior to a benzodiazepine regimen or continued phenobarbital monotherapy. When phenobarbital is utilized as a symptom-triggered monotherapy, a loading dose can be followed by subsequent smaller doses (e.g. 130–260 mg IV, 65 mg PO) until symptoms subside, with a total cumulative dose of over 2–2.5 grams rarely being necessary. As patients approach doses over 2.5 grams they can be prone to additional side effects from phenobarbital, including CNS depression, ataxia, and nystagmus. Due to phenobarbital's various benefits over benzodiazepines, many clinicians prefer utilizing this treatment option.

6.2.3 Adjunctive additional treatments

While GABA-agonist therapy is the mainstay of treatment for AWS, other adjunctive agents may be useful. These medications should only be considered once a patient with AWS has had sufficient GABA-agonist therapy or as an adjunct for safety purposes in the agitated or encephalopathic patient. These adjunctive agents include ketamine, dexmedetomidine, and propofol. Ketamine and propofol are mechanistically therapeutic as ketamine acts as an NMDA receptor antagonist and propofol, like barbiturates, directly stimulates the $GABA_A$ receptor [26]. Dexmedetomidine, a central $alpha_2$ agonist, can be used adjunctively to treat delirium, agitation, but should never be used as a sole, primary agent to treat alcohol withdrawal, as it does not address the underlying physiology. When utilizing dexmedetomidine alone, patients are at risk for decompensating while symptoms are otherwise masked. Airway protection is not necessary for the use of ketamine or dexmedetomidine. While propofol is unnecessary for the patient who is protecting his or her airway, it may be an optimal agent for the intubated patient [18].

Thiamine should also be administered along with concurrent assurance of euglycemia. If patient has no evidence of malabsorption and symptoms are mild to moderate, oral supplementation of 100 mg is sufficient. If any evidence of malabsorption or inability to take medications orally, then thiamine should be given intravenously. If patient is encephalopathic, consider high dose thiamine supplementation out of concern for Wernicke's Encephalopathy or Wernicke-Korsakoff Syndrome (see Complications).

Other than benzodiazepines and barbiturates, there is no role for antiepileptic drugs in treating alcohol withdrawal syndrome or alcohol withdrawal seizures. However, gabapentin may be of some utility in treating the symptoms associated with Post-Acute Withdrawal Syndrome [32]. Upon completion of withdrawal, additional agents, such as naltrexone or acamprosate, should be offered for medication assisted therapy, along with psychosocial and rehabilitative services.

7. Complications and their implications on patient safety

The most important considerations regarding the safety surrounding treating alcohol use disorder and alcohol withdrawal in the hospital setting are early assessment, identification, and intervention and treatment of associated medical complications. Progression of alcohol withdrawal is preventable and delirium tremens is avoidable all together with proper treatment. As patients progress along the AWS spectrum, they become more prone to increasing risk of morbidity and mortality, including sepsis, aspiration, malnutrition, encephalopathy, falls, dysrhythmias, permanent cognitive impairment, and death. Coexisting psychosocial conditions, such as depression and anxiety, should also be attended to decrease risk of self-harm.

Encephalopathy is of particular concern because it is difficult to distinguish and exclude Wernicke's Encephalopathy in the setting of DT. Wernicke's Encephalopathy is about 80% reversible if treated early with high dose thiamine, and if untreated, can progress to Wernicke-Korsakoff Syndrome, which is only about 20% reversible with high dose thiamine. High dose thiamine regimen should be 500 mg IV TID for three days, followed by 100 mg IV or PO for 4 days, followed by 100 mg PO indefinitely. Clinicians should not be tempted to truncate thiamine regimen with improvement of encephalopathy as the observed improvement may be the result of the treatment and, therefore, the full course is indicated.

Interdisciplinary collaboration is of the utmost importance to incorporate expertise in addiction and withdrawal management. Hospitals should invest in these resources for improved patient outcomes. Consultants in this area generally exist in the fields of Addiction Medicine, Addiction Psychiatry, and Medical Toxicology. Case managers and social workers should also be utilized to counsel patients and assist in coordinating further treatment after discharge.

8. Conclusions

In summary, alcohol withdrawal is a complex condition with a wide range of manifestations which results in substantial morbidity and mortality. The underlying pathophysiology of ethanol – chronic GABAergic stimulation – results in a hyperexcitatory state when alcohol withdrawal occurs. Symptoms range from anxiety and tremulousness to seizures, coma, and death. Practitioners should be able to identify patients with AWS risk stratify patients who are at risk of complicated AWS utilizing the various described screening tools. Symptom based assessment tools are also available to guide treatment (CIWA or SEWS). Primary treatment for AWS requires sufficient dosing of GABA agonists (benzodiazepines vs. phenobarbital). Adjunctive therapies also include ketamine and dexmedetomidine, the latter of which should be used cautiously as it does not address the underlying pathophysiology. To ensure patient safety, clinicians should strive to monitor for and prevent known risks and complications associated with AWS. Finally, a multi-disciplinary approach is preferred and should include the expertise of addiction specialists from Addiction Medicine, Addiction Psychiatry, or Medical Toxicology, as well as Case Management.

Author details

Clayton Korson[1] and Thomas Nappe[1,2]*

1 Emergency Department, St. Luke's University Health Network, Bethlehem, PA, United States of America

2 Emergency Department, Medical Toxicology Section, St. Luke's University Health Network, Bethlehem, PA, United States of America

*Address all correspondence to: thomas.nappe@sluhn.org

References

[1] Esser MB, Leung G, Sherk A, et al. Estimated deaths attributable to excessive Alcohol use among US adults aged 20 to 64 years, 2015 to 2019. JAMA Network Open. 2022;**5**(11):e2239485. DOI: 10.1001/jamanetworkopen.2022.39485

[2] Jesse S, Bråthen G, Ferrara M, Keindl M, Ben-Menachem E, Tanasescu R, et al. Alcohol withdrawal syndrome: Mechanisms, manifestations, and management. Acta Neurologica Scandinavica. 2017;**135**:4-16. DOI: 10.1111/ane.12671

[3] National Institute on Alcohol Abuse and Alcoholism. What is A Standard Drink? [Internet]. Available from: https://www.niaaa.nih.gov/alcohols-effects-health/overview-alcohol-consumption/what-standard-drink

[4] Kattimani S, Bharadwaj B. Clinical management of alcohol withdrawal: A systematic review. Industrial Psychiatry Journal. 2013;**22**(2):100-108. DOI: 10.4103/0972-6748.132914

[5] Rogawski MA. Update on the neurobiology of alcohol withdrawal seizures. Epilepsy Currents. 2005;**5**(6):225-230. DOI: 10.1111/j.1535-7511.2005.00071.x

[6] Newman RK, Stobart Gallagher MA, Gomez AE. Alcohol Withdrawal. StatPearls Treasure Island (FL): StatPearls Publishing; 2022 Available from: https://www.ncbi.nlm.nih.gov/books/NBK441882/

[7] Heilig M, Egli M, Crabbe JC, Becker HC. Acute withdrawal, protracted abstinence and negative affect in alcoholism: Are they linked? Addiction Biology. 2010;**15**(2):169-184. DOI: 10.1111/j.1369-1600.2009.00194.x

[8] National Institute on Alcohol Abuse and Alcoholism. Understanding Alcohol Use Disorder [Internet]. Available from: https://www.niaaa.nih.gov/sites/default/files/publications/Alcohol_Use_Disorder_0.pdf

[9] National Institute on Alcohol Abuse and Alcoholism. Screening Tests [Internet]. Available from: https://pubs.niaaa.nih.gov/publications/arh28-2/78-79.htm

[10] Maldonado JR, Sher Y, Ashouri JF, Hills-Evans K, Swendsen H, Lolak S, et al. The "prediction of Alcohol Withdrawal severity scale" (PAWSS): Systematic literature review and pilot study of a new scale for the prediction of complicated alcohol withdrawal syndrome. Alcohol. 2014;**48**(4):375-390. DOI: 10.1016/j.alcohol.2014.01.004

[11] Dyal S, MacLaren R. The assessment and management practices of acute Alcohol Withdrawal: Results of a Nationwide survey of critical care pharmacists. Hospital Pharmacy. 2019;**54**:22-31. DOI: 10.1177/0018578718769241

[12] Maldonado JR, Sher Y, Das S, Hills-Evans K, Frenklach A, Lolak S, et al. Prospective validation study of the prediction of Alcohol Withdrawal severity scale (PAWSS) in medically ill inpatients: A new scale for the prediction of complicated Alcohol Withdrawal syndrome. Alcohol. 2015;**50**(5):509-518. DOI: 10.1093/alcalc/agv043

[13] Sullivan JT, Sykora K, Schneiderman J, Naranjo CA, Sellers EM. Assessment of alcohol withdrawal: The

revised clinical institute withdrawal assessment for alcohol scale (CIWA-Ar). British Journal of Addiction. 1989;**84**(11):1353-1357. DOI: 10.1111/j.1360-0443.1989.tb00737.x

[14] Reoux JP, Miller K. Routine hospital alcohol detoxification practice compared to symptom triggered management with an objective Withdrawal scale (CIWA-Ar). The American Journal on Addictions. 2000 Spring;**9**(2):135-144. DOI: 10.1080/10550490050173208

[15] Beresford T, Anderson M, Pitts B, Learned B, Thumm B, Maravilla F, et al. The severity of ethanol Withdrawal scale in scale-driven Alcohol Withdrawal treatment: A quality assurance study. Alcoholism Treatment Quarterly. 2017;**35**(3):232-242. DOI: 10.1080/07347324.2017.1322418

[16] The American Society of Addiction Medicine Clinical Practice Guideline. Alcohol Withdrawal Management [Internet]. Available from: https://www.asam.org/docs/default-source/quality-science/the_asam_clinical_practice_guideline_on_alcohol-1.pdf?sfvrsn=ba255c2_2

[17] Mirijello A, D'Angelo C, Ferrulli A, Vassallo G, Antonelli M, Caputo F, et al. Identification and management of alcohol withdrawal syndrome. Drugs. 2015;**75**(4):353-365. DOI: 10.1007/s40265-015-0358-1

[18] Long D, Long B, Koyfman A. The emergency medicine management of severe alcohol withdrawal. The American Journal of Emergency Medicine. 2017;**35**(7):1005-1011. DOI: 10.1016/j.ajem.2017.02.002

[19] Schmidt KJ, Doshi MR, Holzhausen JM, Natavio A, Cadiz M, Winegardner JE. Treatment of severe Alcohol Withdrawal. Annals of Pharmacotherapy. 2016;**50**(5):389-401. DOI: 10.1177/1060028016629161

[20] McKeon A, Frye MA, Delanty N. The alcohol withdrawal syndrome. Journal of Neurology, Neurosurgery, and Psychiatry. 2008;**79**(8):854-862. DOI: 10.1136/jnnp.2007.128322

[21] American Psychiatric Association. Delirium Tremens. Diagnostic and statistical manual of mental disorders (5th ed.). 2013. DOI: 10.1176/appi.books.9780890425596

[22] Schuckit MA. Recognition and management of withdrawal delirium (delirium tremens). The New England Journal of Medicine. 2014;**371**(22):2109-2113. DOI: 10.1056/NEJMra1407298

[23] Holbrook AM, Crowther R, Lotter A, Cheng C, King D. Meta-analysis of benzodiazepine use in the treatment of acute alcohol withdrawal. CMAJ. 1999;**160**(5):649-655

[24] Daeppen JB, Gache P, Landry U, Sekera E, Schweizer V, Gloor S, et al. Symptom-triggered vs fixed-schedule doses of benzodiazepine for alcohol withdrawal: A randomized treatment trial. Archives of Internal Medicine. 2002;**162**(10):1117-1121. DOI: 10.1001/archinte.162.10.1117

[25] Muzyk AJ, Leung JG, Nelson S, Embury ER, Jones SR. The role of diazepam loading for the treatment of alcohol withdrawal syndrome in hospitalized patients. The American Journal on Addictions. 2013;**22**(2):113-118. DOI: 10.1111/j.1521-0391.2013.00307.x

[26] Alcohol H, R, Withdrawal. Goldfranks Toxicologic Emergencies. 10th ed. New York, NY: McGraw Hill; 2019

[27] Nisavic M, Nejad SH, Isenberg BM, Bajwa EK, Currier P, Wallace PM,

et al. Use of phenobarbital in Alcohol Withdrawal management - a retrospective comparison study of phenobarbital and benzodiazepines for acute Alcohol Withdrawal Management in General Medical Patients. Psychosomatics. 2019;**60**(5):458-467. DOI: 10.1016/j.psym.2019.02.002

[28] Farkas J. Phenobarbital monotherapy for Alcohol Withdrawal: Simplicity and power. PulmCrit. [Internet]. 2015 Available from: https://emcrit.org/pulmcrit/phenobarbital-monotherapy-for-alcohol-withdrawal-simplicity-and-power/

[29] Gold JA, Rimal B, Nolan A, Nelson L. A strategy of escalating doses of benzodiazepines and phenobarbital administration reduces the need for mechanical ventilation in delirium tremens. Critical Care Medicine. 2007;**35**(3):724-730. DOI: 10.1097/01.CCM.0000256841.28351.80

[30] Rosenson J, Clements C, Simon B, Vieaux J, Graffman S, Vahidnia F, et al. Phenobarbital for acute alcohol withdrawal: A prospective randomized placebo-controlled study. The Journal of Emergency Medicine. 2013;**44**(3):592-8.e2. DOI: 10.1016/j.jemermed.2012.07.056

[31] Oks M, Cleven KL, Healy L, Wei M, Narasimhan M, Mayo PH, et al. The safety and utility of phenobarbital use for the treatment of severe Alcohol Withdrawal syndrome in the medical intensive care unit. Journal of Intensive Care Medicine. 2020;**35**(9):844-850. DOI: 10.1177/0885066618783947

[32] Bahji A, Crockford D, El-Guebaly N. Management of Post-Acute Alcohol Withdrawal: A mixed-studies scoping review. Journal of Studies on Alcohol and Drugs. 2022;**83**(4):470-479

Chapter 7

Patient Safety in the Critical Care Setting: Common Risks and Review of Evidence-Based Mitigation Strategies

Grace M. Arteaga, Lilia Bacu and Pablo Moreno Franco

Abstract

The Intensive Care Unit (ICU) has evolved in the last 50 years. This evolution's main drivers include equipment and software improvements, the patient safety movement, and a better pathophysiological understanding of critical illness. There is mounting pressure from accreditation agencies, governmental regulation, financial challenges, operational dynamics, staffing changes, and increased acuity affecting-ICU care delivery and impacting patient safety. There are higher than ever expectations to improve clinical outcomes after an intensive care stay, to enhance patient safety, to increase family involvement in decision making, and merge the multidisciplinary medical experience into an effective teamwork. Leadership focus is directed towards increasing diversity and inclusion in the workforce while enhancing psychological safety. This review addresses the common risks for patient safety in the intensive care setting and describes the changes in mindset and application of evidence-based mitigation strategies.

Keywords: critical care, safety, ICU, technology, leadership, education, simulation, intensive care

1. Introduction

"First, do no harm", the Hippocratic oath dating back over 2000 years remains the basic philosophy of all healthcare providers caring for patients. Preventing harm in the care of patients has led to a safety culture transformation in the critical care setting [1]. Early studies in adverse events highlighted the role of human factors and organizational systems [2, 3]. The report from the National Academy of Medicine (NAM, formerly Institute of Medicine IOM) "To Err is Human: Building a Safer Health System" [4], described 44,000–98,000 deaths related to medical errors. This report revolutionized the medical system in the United States and shifted the attention towards patient safety. In the general population's mindset, the concept of patient safety has been influenced by the depiction of medical errors in medical television shows [5] and the news media [6, 7]. Intensive care is an area where safe practice is of paramount importance. Errors have been reported in intensive care units (ICUs) worldwide commonly associated with medication related events, indwelling lines, airway specific, and equipment failure [8]. Patients with organ failure or with a requirement for a higher intensity of care have elevated odds for exposure to a significant event [9].

The Agency for Healthcare Research and Quality (AHRQ), an official website of the Department of Health and Human Services in the Unites States, defines errors as "acts of commission or omission leading to an undesirable outcome or significant potential for such an outcome" [10]. Adverse events are defined as "any injury caused by medical care" and do not imply negligence, poor quality care, or error [10]. An adverse event can be associated with an unfavorable clinical outcome related to any part of a diagnosis or therapy (known complications), or not related to the disease process (e.g., pneumothorax after a central line placement). Medical errors are considered the third leading cause of death in the US [11]. After 20 years of effort in improving patient safety, there is a better foundation to address potential solutions using evidence-based approaches across institutions involving multiple work units. Evolving health care to become a High-Reliability Organization (HRO) is a constant journey to excellence. It requires a transformation where leadership is committed to engaging in patient safety solutions at the work unit level, to evolve into a culture of safety, and support advanced performance improvement methodology [12].

The objective of this review is to (1) summarize the current view of patient safety in the critically ill patient setting and (2) highlight novel approaches to improve safety in critical care.

1.1 Method

1.1.1 Search strategy

The information included in this review was obtained from a search conducted using PubMed, MEDLINE, and Google to access government publications and industry related websites. Single and paired combination of terms included patient safety, critical care, intensive care, simulation, telemedicine, medical error, adverse events, psychological safety, post intensive care syndrome, leadership, technology, education, culture of safety, teamwork, COVID-19, shared-decision making, artificial intelligence, communication, interprofessional collaboration, checklist, and bundle of care. The themes extracted from this process were discussed between the authors and with professional colleagues with expertise in patient safety and served as the foundation for important topics related to patient safety and critical care.

1.2 Critical care safety events

From the number of events reported by the Office of Inspector General (OIG) in 2010, a global 27% of Medicare patients experienced harm events [13]; while 25% experienced harm in 2018 (with 13.1% experiencing an adverse event that resulted in patient harm, defined as an event that requires intervention but does not result in permanent harm) [14]. These two reports also demonstrated that after a physician review of these events, 44% of them were deemed clearly or likely preventable in 2010, compared to the most recent report in 2022 where 43% were determined to be preventable.

The critical care setting holds a number of patient safety challenges related to the complexity and intensity of care [9], the high-risk decision making in clinically unstable patients [15], and the LOS in an ICU setting [16, 17]. Adverse drug events

(ADEs) result in more than half a million injuries or deaths in U.S. hospitalized patients in intensive care units [18]. The adult critical care literature has reported significant variability of adverse events in the intensive care unit (ICU), ranging from 0.8 adverse events and 1.5 serious errors for a 10-bed critical care unit [19] to 1.7 error per patient per day in a medical-surgical of a university hospital [20]. A more recent systematic review and meta-analysis demonstrated a significant increase in ICU and hospital length of stay (LOS) in patients who suffered an adverse event [21]. In this systematic review, the authors were not able to establish a strong relationship between safety events and mortality, possibly related to patient heterogeneity. However, in a prospective clinical study performed in 70 French ICUs, it was reported that having more than two adverse events increased the risk of death [22]. This group was able to determine that those patients with more severe illness were at higher risk for an adverse event.

The pediatric population in ICU is not precluded from suffering adverse events. Medication errors are frequent, particularly in the younger group [17] and are considered preventable adverse events. Dosing errors are reported as the most common subtype. Pediatric medications are calculated based on weight or BMI and usually include a fraction of an adult dose, augmenting the potential for a 10-fold dosing errors [23]. A more recent study addressed human factors as contributing to prescription errors in pediatric intensive care units (PICUs) and found that cognitive burden, both physical (fatigue, distraction) and psychological (workload change, inexperience) were the most common latent factors associated to these findings [24].

Capturing and measuring adverse events challenges the incidence and mortality statistics related to unintentional medical errors. The development and implementation of incident reporting systems in healthcare has become a fundamental strategy aiming at improving patient safety [25]. Despite the success of reporting "near misses" or "close calls" in the aviation and nuclear plant industry, underreporting has become a factor undermining incident reporting within the medical system [26]. Several factors affecting incident reporting in healthcare include fear of adverse consequences and ineffective processes/systems of reporting [27]. In critical care, both adult and pediatric, factors associated to increased reporting include anonymity, regular feedback about errors reported and solution implementation, and a healthy culture of safety [28]. Other efforts to collect reliable data within the medical system include the development of a group of quality indicators by the Agency for Healthcare Research and Quality (AHRQ) [29] in an attempt to nationally provide a measure to monitor performance overtime and apply the information collected to the development of solutions targeting error prevention. The institution of global triggers became available through the Institute for Healthcare Improvement (IHI) [30] and was designed to provide a method for accurate identification of adverse events and rate measurement of these events overtime. A hospitalized standardized mortality ratio (HSMR) was implemented in the United Kingdom in 2001 [31].

1.3 Socioeconomic impact

For any given year, the cost of adverse events to the American health system can be measured in the billions of dollars. In 2008, an OIG report stated the cost was $324 million for the single month of October 2008 [13]. In the 2022 OIG report, an extra Medicare cost was incurred for all preventable and nonpreventable events. This report calculated hundreds of millions of dollars for October 2018 [14]. In 2006, Jain et al. demonstrated that the use of quality improvement initiatives directed to enhance the culture of safety and teamwork, with the specific goal to decrease hospital acquired infections, led to a 21% reduction in cost per ICU discharge [32]. Adopting bundles of care, the authors demonstrated a decline in ventilator associated pneumonia, bloodstream infection, and urinary tract infection, and the number of adverse events decreased from an average of 25 events per day to less than 5. The creation and adoption of ICU bundles of care for adults [33] and pediatric populations [34] have provided a new practice model for liberating critically ill patients from the ICU environment. The strategic implementation of bundles of care leads to a reduction in hospital cost [35].

The indirect cost related to ICU events is considered of significant magnitude. Intensive care survivors reported suffering from physical, cognitive, or mental health symptoms long after dismissal from their ICU stay [36]. Evidence recognizes that longer ICU delirium is associated with increased cognitive deficits [37]. As a result, the Society of Critical Care Medicine coined the term post-intensive care syndrome (PICS) and addressed strategies to mitigate unfavorable outcomes [38]. Compelling research notes that this phenomenon is pertinent to all ages, children included. The pediatric recovery trajectory affects the patient and the family nucleus in the long-term and has not been fully elucidated [39]. Further, families of ICU survivors also demonstrate psychiatric diagnoses, including depression, posttraumatic stress disorder, anxiety, and complicated grief [38]. The cognitive impairment and psychiatric diagnosis lead to an economic impact because of loss of income from the patient or the caregiver [40]. The future of critical care is shifting towards the ICU survivorship and their successful rehabilitation [41].

The human impact of adverse events directly affects the well-being of patients (first victim). Similarly, healthcare providers (second victim) are negatively affected [42, 43] eliciting emotional distress characterized by guilt, anxiety, remorse, depression, burnout, and physical symptoms ranging from fatigue to sleep disturbances [44]. A high rate of adverse medication events occur in the critical care setting [18] with greater harm to the patient when compared to non-ICU populations [45]. The consequences on the well-being of the healthcare provider in the critical care setting after a medical error occurs result in personal blame and guilt [46].

2. Causality

The patient safety movement has significantly shifted from attempting to prevent errors to decreasing harm to the patient [47]. Focusing on minimizing or preventing harm draws attention to the environment and processes. A systematic approach to assessing the quality of care includes defining the objectives for review and the processes within the organization that interact with the human factors. In approaching quality of care assessment, the Donabedian triad [48] classifies three categories: Structure-Process-Outcome (**Figure 1**) as an effort to improve the quality of care provided. In this model, harm can be seen as an outcome, while errors are approached with a magnifying lens. This approach avoids focusing on the provider's responsibility for harm, and advocates orienting towards the system involved in the error, knowing that errors and harm are not always linked. A mature culture of safety leads to injury prevention by asking "why" during every step of the root cause analysis and by supporting the development of an injury prevention model [49]. It also provides a more constructive follow-up to families and patients, as evidenced by a decrease in the number of claims by half, associated reductions in legal fees, less cost per claim and decreased settlement amount when changes in the response to harm with a

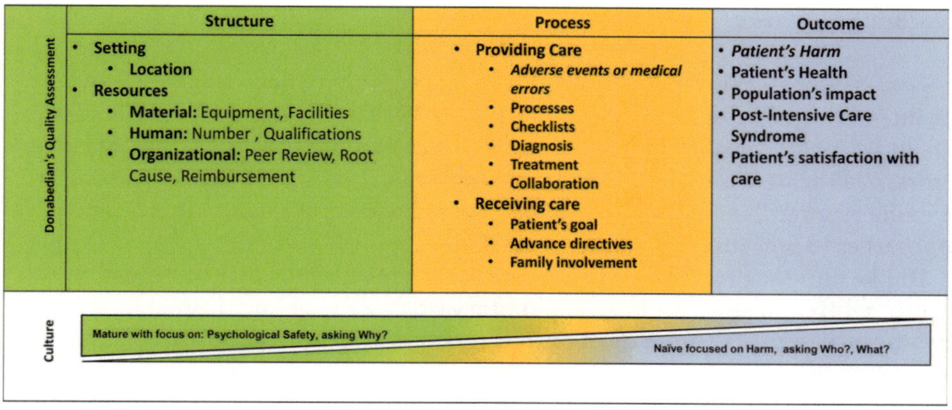

Figure 1.
Relationship between Donabedian's quality assessment model and culture. Donabedian's Quality Assessment integrated with the Culture of Safety. The beginning of a cultural model of quality improvement assessment can shift between focusing on an outcome to focusing on the structure within an ecosystem. The elements that Donabedian labeled in this quality assessment model are described along with a culture of safety stage of development. As the culture evolves, the attention is re-directed towards the process of care and common improvement activities are directed to reduce variation. At a mature level, the culture of safety focuses the solutions to system re-engineering and psychological safety (Figure based on Donabedian A. The Quality of Care. How can it be assessed? Jama 1988;12:1743).

communication and optimal resolution approach is implemented [50–52]. A mature culture of safety focuses on the system and the impact on people, elevating psychological safety, concentrating on why the event occurred within that environment; and why the established redundancies within the system were not effective in aborting the event. Changing the culture of safety where the outcome (harm) is not the center of the investigation to one where the investigative questions move away from what happened and who was involved, increases the trust in the evaluation process and decreases the fear of participating in the event assessment [53]. Emphasizing on the individual participants and not the system assessment results in further degradation of the culture, prevents people from speaking up, and leads to more cover-ups due to concerns of being labeled as incompetent as well as enhances the fear of retaliation.

2.1 Intensive care and teamwork

An effective and efficient workload involves a highly specialized workforce where teamwork is the central process [54]. The intensive care unit is a highly complex system where the most acute and severe medical cases are cared for in the acute and chronic phases. The complexity includes the highly technological support with continuous assessment and integration of multiple disciplines in the decision-making process [55]. Collaboration, coordination, and networking between disciplines aim to achieve the same goal, patient care, and better patient outcomes [54]. The type of teamwork described in the intensive care unit is commonly characterized as multidisciplinary, although other terms such as interdisciplinary, multi-professional, and interprofessional have also been used [56]. For this chapter, we will use the term interprofessional collaboration [57]. In addition, when the patient and family members are included in the decision-making process, the effects of stressful decisions among parents are mitigated, the sense of remorse is lessened [58] and the levels of dissatisfaction among family members is reduced [59].

2.2 Common errors

Non-diagnostic medical errors and adverse events have been well described in the intensive care setting, impacting hospital LOS and ICU days [21]. The common categories include medication errors, communication and handoff errors, teamwork errors, healthcare-associated infections, and surgical errors. All these areas can be easily reported, investigated, and have been the focus of quality improvement approaches to prevent and minimize harm.

Unlike non-diagnostic errors that are easier to investigate, diagnostic errors require a different strategy. In an exploratory study delving into diagnostic errors, Barwise et al. found that the most cited errors across different ICU stakeholder groups include: a) difficulties associated with organizational factors, such as availability and relevance of the information within the electronic health record (EHR), workflow problems and capacity issues; b) difficulties related to interpersonal factors, e.g., poor communication, failed handoff, and suboptimal teamwork; and c) difficulties related to the individual clinician or patient factors [60].

A systematic review in Pediatric Critical Care found that up to 67% of diagnostic errors in the pediatric critical care setting are related to system factors, while up to 30% included cognitive factors. Notably, 40% of the diagnostic errors combined cognitive and system factors [61].

As the field of patient safety has evolved through the years, diagnostic errors have become an important area of investigation. A superficial view of this topic might target only the provider who, based on skill and experience, reached a medical decision [62]. However, considering our current scope and development of evidence in patient safety, a deeper understanding of decision-making leads to scrutinizing the institutional structure and processes available, including technical and human factors, policies and procedures, and a culture of harm prevention [63]. Whether building safety checks into the healthcare system will suffice to prevent diagnostic errors is yet to be determined.

2.3 Taxonomy

The Agency for Healthcare Research and Quality (AHRQ) and the Patient Safety Network (PSNET) define near-miss events as "errors that occur in the process of providing medical care that are detected and corrected before a patient is harmed." They have also been called "close calls" [10]. In the current complex ICU environment, identifying and correcting events before they reach the patient is paramount as healthcare organizations engage in the care delivery process in critical care environments. To help us understand this undertaking, James Reasons's Swiss cheese model illustrates how small but multiple systems' failures lead to safety events which are often harmful to patients [30]. Within the glossary of patient safety terminology relevant to this review, we include "sentinel events" and "never events". The AHRQ notes that "sentinel events", a term utilized by The Joint Commission, can also be viewed as "never events" and it further defines sentinel events as "an unexpected occurrence involving death or serious physiological or psychological injury, or the risk thereof" [64] which highlights the interchangeable aspect of this important terminology [65]. A common taxonomy for event classification widely used in publications and at institutional levels was designed by the National Coordinating Council for Medication Error Reporting and Prevention (NCC MERP). In this index, errors are graded in categories A through I, depending on the level of harm (**Figure 2**) [66].

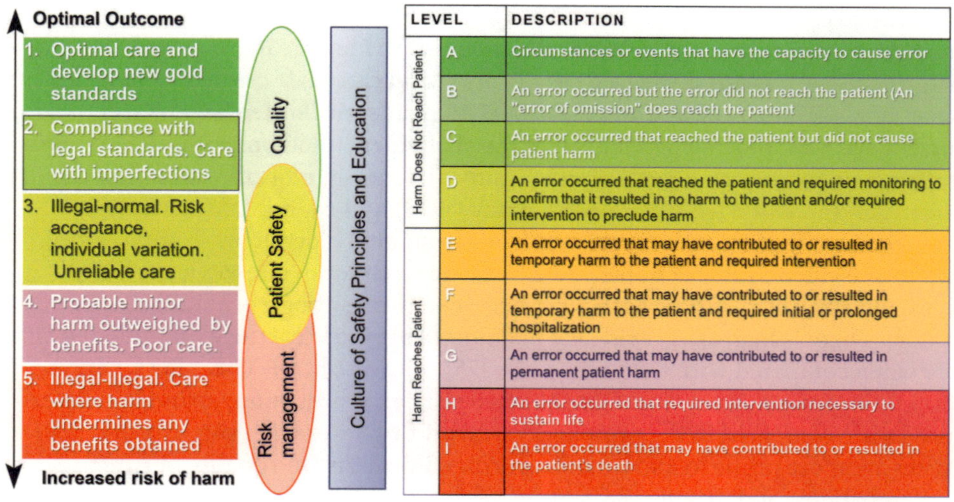

Figure 2.
*Coordination between quality improvement, patient safety and risk management using culture of safety principles to predict, prevent and manage harm. A quality oversight team must organize the response to all events being reported, independently of the level. The most serious events will require risk management to engage and deploy resources to perform a Root-Cause-Analysis. Less severe events, such as near-misses, can be managed by the Patient Safety and Quality office, ultimately responsible for developing standards of optimal care, new gold standards, ensuring compliance with established policies and procedures. It is everyone's responsibility to create a culture of safety and to generate the educational tools to predict, prevent and manage harm. (*Permission is hereby granted to reproduce information contained herein provided that such reproduction shall not modify the text and shall include the copyright notice).*

Severe error investigations commonly involve the root cause analysis (RCA) process developed by the Joint Commission on Accreditation of Healthcare Organizations. A widely used approach to categorizing the root cause of errors was published by Charles Vincent [67] and continues to be helpful in event investigations. It follows a similar logic as the Swiss cheese model created after James Reason's publication on latent human failures [68], emphasizing that the analyses of medical errors should anchor on diving into root causes that explain decision making, not on the whom and how, but in the why. The goal is to identify the gaps within the ecosystem using root cause analyses to address the system's failures. This recommendation aligns with The Joint Commission's® goal of zero harm. Ideally, investigating near misses can identify gaps requiring proactive intervention. Near miss reporting is weak unless it is closely associated to a negative outcome [69]. These types of events are rarely reported as they are time-consuming and require additional evaluative effort. Furthermore, it is challenging to measure their results. As we move towards a preventative rather than reactive approach healthcare, exploring the near-miss events should be a gold standard.

2.4 Staffing impact, coronavirus disease 2019 (COVID-19) era and current challenges

The COVID 19 pandemic spurred on a mass workforce exodus from healthcare and increasing emotional distress, impacting all levels of care across the healthcare continuum, including the critical care environment [70]. Considering this new phenomenon, organizations were forced to reimagine innovative ICU care models [71], recognizing that the ICU of the future will have a different team composition with varied operational strategies [72]. The ongoing challenge healthcare institutions encounter is the increasing number of patients with life-threatening conditions in critical care settings. A decreased supply of critical care staff created from a "deficit status quo" [73] and the additional COVID-19 pandemic burden have exacerbated the current systems, putting patient safety at risk. Evidence demonstrates that nursing staffing and workload in the ICU have a direct impact on mortality rates, nosocomial infections, increased length of hospital stay (LOS) and overall inferior nursing performance [74]. The COVID 19 pandemic prompted older generations to retire, mothers decided to stay at home and care for their children due to a lack of available childcare, while others decided to leave healthcare altogether and pursue other careers. There is increasing evidence that nurses plan to leave the workforce at a faster rate when compared with the past decade [75]. As a result, the Great Resignation shifted the predominant workforce characteristics towards younger and less experienced staff compared to the pre-pandemic workforce. Research suggests that novice nurses are more prone to make medical errors, impacting the quality of care provided to their patients and driving the healthcare community to search for innovative approaches in education and clinical practice [76]. Younger generations prefer collaboration over competition and mentorship relationships with their bosses over the standard hierarchical structures in healthcare organizations [77]. This preference can be harnessed to drive patient safety initiatives in critical care while helping co-create new collaboration models.

This technology-savvy workforce also demands more sophisticated hardware and software that enables their professional responsibilities. Modernizing, enhancing, and automating processes and integrating systems that improve the ICU workflows will be crucial to retaining the current workforce.

Understanding the needs of the current workforce will help organizations develop retention strategies, create an enjoyable work environment, and subsequently improve patient safety. Intangibles such as job structures that can maintain a better work-life balance, burnout prevention, and joy creation will be non-negotiable.

3. Mitigation strategies and proposed solutions

3.1 Culture of safety

Institutional Core Values: At an institutional level, the quality oversight team must create a cultural shift by coordinating that each department addresses safety, process improvement, professional outcome assessment, and patient satisfaction. This cultural shift should be focused on personal responsibility and behaviors consistent with institutional core values [1, 32, 78].

3.2 Decision making

All healthcare providers who attend to patients in the medical system are highly motivated, highly trained individuals whose professional goal is to support others in their most vulnerable moments. It is therefore of the utmost importance to approach medical errors from a systems perspective, understanding that human decision-making is anchored in an evolving medical system where ideally, patient safety should depend on error anticipation and prevention [47]. HROs e.g., nuclear power industry, commercial aviation, aeronautics, base their safety on organized algorithms. Humans are placed in an environment where decision-making is anticipated, and the appropriate tools exist to minimize risk (e.g., checklists).

Little attention has been given to a type of medical error that is difficult to measure and rarely reported: diagnostic errors. This group of errors have been recognized as a significant patient safety threat, involving intra- and inter-professional teamwork [79, 80]. In 2015, the National Academies of Sciences (NAM) released a landmark report addressing this concern: Improving Diagnosis in Health Care [81]. Decision-making and subsequent actions for diagnostic and treatment purposes occur in an ecosystem that involves structure, processes, policies, and an accepted culture within an institution. It is imperative to understand diagnostic reasoning and critical thinking to improve diagnostic performance and reduce error.

Daniel Kahneman won a Nobel Prize in 1982 for the systematic identification and characterization of human decision behaviors which were not previously described. His book, *Thinking, Fast and Slow*, describes two cognitive systems of thinking and decision making: System 1 or Type 1 (automatic, emotional, stereotypic, unconscious), and System 2 or Type 2 (slow, effortful, infrequent, logical, calculating, conscious) [82]. He theorized that System 1 uses cognitive "shortcuts" (heuristics) to reduce the cognitive cost of decision-making. In this area, cognitive biases can preclude the bayesian approach to medical decisions. Cognitive psychologists have explored medical reasoning, the use of these mental systems, and cognitive self-monitoring strategies (metacognition, debiasing) that allow for a mental pause to recognize and shift between these processes [83, 84]. Understanding cognitive decision-making processes that influence medical decision behavior will impact cognitive errors. Education in cognitive science and critical thinking, associated with metacognitive skill training [85] using curricula can provide practitioners with the tools to understand and recognize cognitive biases, particularly in high-paced, high-risk specialties such as Anesthesiology, Critical Care, and Emergency Medicine [86].

4. Leadership

4.1 Leading with humility

Leading with humility is an attribute sought after in healthcare, mainly because most subject matter experts undergo rigorous training and become highly skilled before being able to treat and manage critically ill patients. Bringing these experts together and capturing the collective genius requires humble leadership, collaboration, and a shared purpose: to produce safety outcomes. Owens et al. proposed several characteristics of leader humility: "(a) a manifested willingness to view oneself accurately, (b) an appreciation of others' strengths and contributions, and (c) teachability or openness to new ideas and feedback" [87]. Leading with humility is a signature trait [88] of inclusive leadership characterized by humble inquiry. Considering the fast-paced environment of our current ICUs and the commitment to patient safety, servant leadership is key to being open to asking the questions to which we do not know the answers. Centering the message around the patient, we recognize the importance of leading with humility.

4.2 Inclusion

The current volatile, unpredictable, complex, and ambiguous healthcare environment suggests that everyone's voice can be mission-critical [89]. This can be accomplished if we cultivate inclusive and agile leadership. In this climate, inclusive leadership is crucial to collaboration and the avoidance of preventable failures. ICU teams' structure involves physician attendings, residents, nurses, respiratory therapists, advanced practice providers and many other roles from diverse backgrounds.

Empirical evidence continues to grow about the importance of inclusive leadership and its influence on culture in healthcare. The *Leadership Saves Lives* study demonstrated that organizational culture and performance improvement significantly influence mortality rates for patients experiencing acute myocardial infarction [90]. Inclusive leadership crosses hierarchies and invites distinct perspectives and authentic participation. This helps build trust among peers, psychological safety, and situational humility. For example, when physician leaders of intensive care units invite dialog on "what else can we do; how can we tackle this opportunity together," they demonstrate openness to other ideas and foster collaborative problem-solving. Inclusion leads to greater engagement, team performance, and improved patient outcomes [91]. The care for our critically ill patients has become increasingly complex, and teams rely on each other to save lives.

4.3 Psychological safety

Psychological safety is foundational to healthcare organizations and the conduit through which patient safety occurs. This phenomenon and its related antecedent concepts have been studied since the 1990s, with much progress made in recent years. It has been linked to team performance [92], ethical conduct [93], team diversity [94, 95], incivility [96], reporting of medical errors [94], innovation [97], and has been identified as a predictor for turnover intent [98]. A great problem occurs when medical errors are not reported due to lower psychological safety. The organization and patients suffer as a result, either through direct harm or missed opportunities to prevent latent failures.

Compelling evidence shows that when team members speak up, they are willing and able to talk about mistakes, collectively tackle improvement, and are more likely to innovate and drive solutions [91]. Nembhard and Edmondson discovered that intensive care units which foster high levels of psychological safety spontaneously decreased morbidity and mortality without additional interventions such as training or education. Despite growing evidence, psychological safety in healthcare organizations remains an untapped opportunity. Some factors include unmitigated and unapologetic hierarchies, fear of endangering someone's life, and old authoritarian leadership models. Fostering psychological safety in the current complex environment is crucial for catching near misses [69], addressing medical errors, and continuously learning from them.

High psychological safety is a prerequisite to advancing patient safety. Over the years, research in social psychology has identified humble inquiry as the avenue to build psychological safety. Recent data shows that leaders can effectively build it not only through seeking feedback from team members, but also by sharing criticism they previously received, and by being openly vulnerable. Grant and Coutifaris randomly assigned leaders to criticize themselves as opposed to asking for criticism. Just inviting them to do that once, it increased psychological safety in their teams for at least a year [99]. This led teams to organize monthly vulnerability meetings and reserve time for "check-ins" on what needs to improve. Other structured practices that enable and support psychological safety include time outs, huddles, debriefs, listening and communication as agreed upon competencies, understood method to raise a concern or question, and escalation protocols.

5. Technology

Unfortunately, even in modern medicine, with some of the most advanced medical equipment in the world, it is not an easy task to be able to remove noise, recognize a deteriorating patient in early stages, initiate timely resuscitation maneuvers, correctly identify a differential diagnosis, and orchestrate highly complex multidisciplinary teams to focus on critical short term goals while maintaining a strategic plan to allow the "person-in-the-bed" to recover to a high functioning level, as close as possible to the pre-morbid state and prevent a possible PICS.

Because the ICU is only one segment in the patient's journey, we must be comfortable stepping outside the physical boundaries and create operating conditions that include electronic outreach and monitoring in a control tower fashion, proactive ICU nursing rounding, and rapid response, preventing complications of medical care, enhanced rehabilitation pathways, avoiding transition of care gaps, preparing survivor clinics, readmission prevention with advance care at home, and others yet to be invented.

5.1 Smart alerts

Changing the ICU framework towards early identification and protocolized management of critically ill patients is perhaps one of the most significant contributions developed in recent years [100]. ICU and Quality Improvement teams participate in local, national, and international research teams to develop processes and decision support tools deployed at the point of care in critically ill patients [101, 102]. Evidence supports that smart alerts improve the care provided in the ICU, some examples include: (a) adherence to basic critical care processes such as the sepsis bundle [103], (b) ventilator bundle with sedation holiday compliance [100, 101], and (c) enhanced risk stratification utilizing severity of disease score calculators [104].

When smart alerts are deliberately deployed using implementation science tools, they can lead to better outcomes such as decreased in ICU, hospital, and 28 days mortality rates from sepsis [103] and alleviated cognitive workload with more accessible navigation through the EMR [105]. Smart alerts also have the potential to add value in intensive care units by lowering cost, decreasing ICU and Hospital LOS, improving disability-adjusted life years, quality-adjusted life years, and incremental cost-effectiveness ratio [106].

To juxtapose the attributes smart alerts have, they can potentiate negative consequences if the alerts are missed or delayed due to technical difficulties, which might translate into delays in care. Some examples include technical failures, firewall blocking, and security issues with smartphone/tablet alert delivery which may present a barrier to optimal alert delivery in the ICU setting [100].

End-user fatigue contributes to disengagement with the alerting mechanisms; it increases human error, information overload, as well as alerts with higher false positive (noise) rates. This can derive from user preferences for specific alert delivery methods, which can affect compliance [107].

5.2 Decision support systems and artificial intelligence

Artificial Intelligence (AI) tools intended for practice enhancement will have to address these challenges. Based on insights gained from studies of human error [60], understanding of information needs [108], and both cognitive and organizational ergonomics [109], we need to establish an infrastructure to develop and test advanced analytics centered on clinician's needs and ICU decision support tools applicable both at the bedside and across the hospital of the future. AI applications in critical care are in the early stages of development. Some of the initially published studies showcase applications to predict LOS, ICU readmission, mortality rates, and early identification of complications and risk stratification [110]. The promise of AI enhancing safety in the ICU depends on its successful application to common ICU problems such as point-of-care ultrasound, volume assessment, medication titration, ventilator management, and other smart devices [111]. An essential element to consider when evaluating the role of AI is that scientific evidence still needs to catch up with machine learning algorithms. For example, the FDA has approved 130 AI devices, of which 126 were based only on retrospective research [112]. Also, we must ensure that measures are taken to avoid algorithmic biases such as race, gender, and other social determinants of health. As such, algorithm developers should transparently report the steps taken for the algorithm to be equitable and representative of the entire population or at least report the specific input data sources, population composition, bias assessment validation, and training data location and period [112].

The role of AI-based technologies in critical care is expanding exponentially. Much of the work utilizing AI in intensive care has been around predictive analytics for early identification of deteriorating/at risk patients and machine learning models to predict patient's clinical trajectory [111]. Solutions such as using predictive analytics to provide early insights on whether a patient will develop delirium [113], pressure injuries [114] from prolonged ICU stay, sepsis [115], or have unattended bed exits triggering falls, have the potential to become the gold standard for the healthcare industry. They augment the decision support process, enhance reliability, and accelerate much-needed agility in critical care. These tools are crucial to optimizing the care our patients receive and achieving the goal of zero harm. Halamka and Cerrato describe in *The Digital Reconstruction of Healthcare* that the future belongs to advanced data analytics. Supporting human skills with Big Data and AI-based algorithms can be equated to "giving the best artists the best analytic tools" [116]. It will elevate the potential for decreased ICU stay, and fewer hospital-acquired infections, among many other healthcare-associated conditions. This vision advances the frontiers of patient safety into an ultra-safe space. Another promising feature of AI-based solutions is solidifying healthcare in the high-reliability space where there is less dependence on human behavior and more reliance on systems and structures. Minimizing patient harm while delivering care includes high-reliability practices which lead to a "more integrated picture of operations at the moment and earlier detection of potential threats to safety" [117]. Empirical evidence suggests that advanced predictive analytics must be part of the solution to improve the patient's safety journey in critical care environments.

5.3 Electronic medical record (EMR)

The transition from handwritten records to EMR has improved efficiency, revenue capture, and billing. Evidence supports using EMRs to enhance patient safety and improve outcomes [118]. Reports exist promoting that EMR saves time during documentation [119]. If critical elements of EMR design and implementation are overlooked, then the positive or negative impact on patient safety and quality could potentially be amplified [108]. To appropriately design and implement an EMR in the ICU, crucial elements must be considered, including information overload, clinical setting, rule development, controlled environment testing, field testing, and implementation science. As an example, Pickering et al. have demonstrated that after following these steps for introducing a novel Ambient Warning Response and Evaluation (AWARE), EMR was associated with improved efficiency of data access and decreased cognitive overload due to improved presentation format [120].

5.4 Dashboards and feedback

The amount of information and metrics being tracked by ICU providers and leaders can be overwhelming. It is paramount that critical priorities are distilled at the unit, team, and provider levels. Priorities need to be divided into metrics to induce improvements that can be tracked in dashboards and transparently published and accessed. To sustain the gains, providers should be given factual and non-judgmental feedback as close to real-time as possible. Utilizing this methodology with the sepsis care bundle compliance, for example, some ICUs have been able to improve compliance, [121] sustain gains, and translate them into improved patient outcomes [103, 122].

6. Education

The critical care setting is a highly technical, fast-pacing, high-risk clinical area where medical knowledge advancement requires frequent up-to-date resources, and skill mastering involves the confidence and expertise of team members at different levels. Novice healthcare providers need the experience in critical thinking and skill mastering commonly provided within the practice, arguably impinging on patient safety principles. The balance between autonomy and supervision in all disciplines is an ever-changing part of daily practice in the intensive care unit. The challenges in an increased demand on training hours, limited patient encounters, and the focus on patient safety have led to relying more on innovation and technology to provide an effective curriculum.

Recognizing the degree of safety within the critical care practice can set the stage to determine the priorities needed in education. Education is frequently embedded within practice to maintain a high level of patient safety and minimize harm. **Figure 3** describes the functional levels frequently found in this setting, including the unique nature of the ICU, where teams often move within a spectrum of an ultra-safe activity to an ultra-adaptive activity, setting the stage for a higher risk for errors [123].

Medical simulation has been introduced as an effective methodology in medical education in general [124]; and within the critical care practice to impart critical care principles, particularly in skill acquisition and competence [125]. This technology has had a widely positive educational impact on all health-related professional groups [126]. It provides significant results when combined with reflective debriefing, considered the most crucial component in healthcare simulation [127]. The interactive, bidirectional, and reflective conversation at the end of a simulation exercise cements the basis of adult learning strategies using experiential learning. Several methodologies have been described in the literature, including debrief timing, methodology, structure alternatives, and process elements. The facilitator-guided debrief is the most common methodology and improves individual and team performance [128]. Recently, a more positive approach to debrief, learning from success (LFS), has been endorsed where adaptation is the focus of the exercise with a scenario that includes unanticipated and problematic disruptions that are presented to the learners [129]. Faculty members using the LFS approach require a deeper understanding of human factor science, patient safety, implementation science, and organizational psychology.

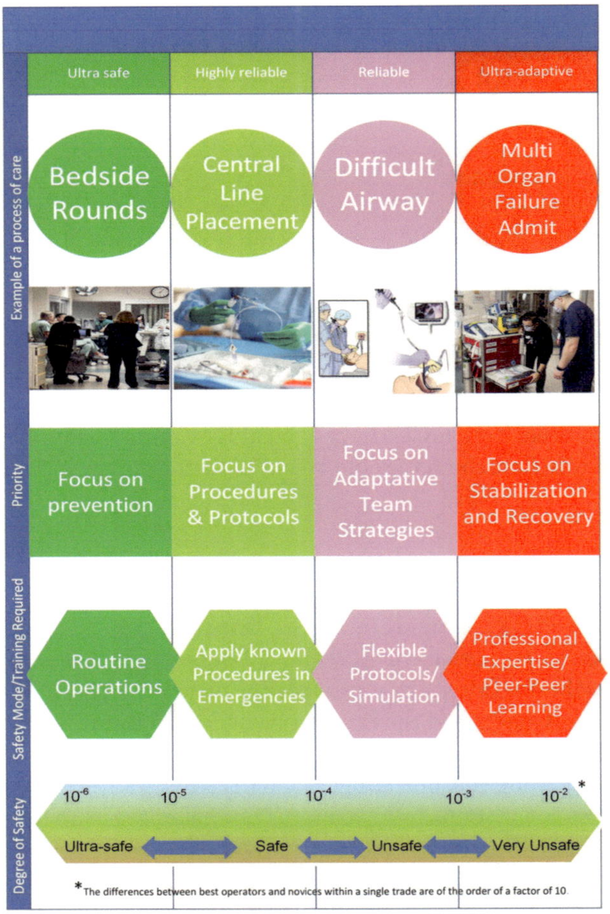

Figure 3.
*Approaches to safety education and practice in the intensive care unit. Successful Critical Care practices feel comfortable with fast changes in pace and complexity. These changes come with an increase in risk, translating into variations in safety levels for decisions and procedures executed. ICU conditions can change very quickly ranging between an ultra-safe environment as in bedside rounds, a highly reliable as in central line placement, a reliable as in difficult airways or an ultra-adaptive in multiorgan failure/code situations. With this construct in mind, education should be directed to arm providers with the tools to think fast and slow between: routine operations/focus on prevention, applying known procedures in emergencies/focus on protocols, being flexible/focus on adaptative team strategies and professional expertise/focus on stabilization followed by recovery. *(Vincent, C and R. Amalberti, Strategies for the Real World 2015, Chapter 3, pg 31. Ref. 123).*

Can the use of medical simulation improve the goals of patient safety and decrease harm to patients? The current body of literature describes enhanced skills and knowledge, competence, better outcomes, and lower error rates using procedural simulation training [130]. The use of simulation has also been applied to hospital design to identify latent conditions and mitigate safety concerns in a systematic process [131].

6.1 Skills development and assessment

The skill set required for the ICU healthcare providers is unique and differentiated from other work units within the hospital. Some of these skills include high risk airway management, conscious sedation, management of mechanical ventilatory and circulatory support, among others. There are several ways to ensure providers who join the ICU have the necessary skill set for critical decision-making and advanced procedures. Standard credentialing processes and certification have been established to ensure providers complete a certain number of procedures. It is essential to recognize the limitations of relying narrowly on procedural skills when ICU leadership makes hiring decisions. Having mechanisms to evaluate soft skills and decision-making prior to hiring can enhance safety by elevating the starting skillset. One tool to consider is using simulation scenarios that mimic typical decompensation events to evaluate and optimize performance. Utilizing simulation center-based interviews for nurse practitioners and physician assistants at one institution improved retention. It also decreased actions for practice deficiencies compared to a conventional interview method [132].

6.1.1 Cultural values

When new employees join, they only have a basic understanding of the organization based on small bits of information gathered during the interview process. During their onboarding, we need to establish a memorable experience that helps them internalize the expectations, including service values, cultural components, [78] shared understanding of how we work, how we interact, fair and just culture, and how we respond to safety events and improvement culture.

6.1.2 Defining successful ICU outcomes

Meaningful outcomes must be concordant with the patient's wishes. From the patient's perspective, the quality of life, independence, and quality of death and dying are often more important than survival per se. We also must prevent catastrophic long-term consequences for patients and their families, many of which are iatrogenic.

6.2 Shared-decision making

Informed Medical Decisions Foundation defines shared decision-making as "Shared decision-making is a collaborative process that allows patients, or their surrogates, and clinicians to make health care decisions together, taking into account the best scientific evidence available, as well as the patient's values, goals, and preferences" [133]. Subsequently, effective communication with patients and families is the pillar of shared decision-making and patient-centered care [134]. The availability of health information technology (HIT) allows for increased connectivity between patients and providers. A systematic review of the current literature addressing patient access to their EMR, reported increased patient engagement with the medical system, increased communication with their health care teams, increased discovery of medical errors, and improved adherence to medication [135]. Furhermore, vast research conducted in the shared decisiom-making space, clarified the opportunities related to patient's preferences, goals and values, especially in the ICU setting where requests for futile interventions often arise [136]. From the patient and family's perspective, effective communication enhances trust in their healthcare providers and improves the perception of their care within a system [137–139].

7. Professional development

Patient safety science continues to be an ever-changing field in health care. Continuous professional development in all disciplines and lifelong learning are essential to meeting patients' expectations, regulatory requirements, personal growth, and job satisfaction. An integral part of the development and organization of a safety program within an institution is continuing professional development. This requires a well-developed systematic approach to individual and team growth, in conjunction with technology implementation and invariably uses principles of human-engineering science. Enhancing communication between professionals, various services, and with patients requires leadership involvement in creating an environment of excellence [55].

8. Team dynamics

The relevance of team training is evident in the critical care setting. On any given day, various disciplines and providers from different professions interact to provide the best care to critically ill patients. This fluid interaction is significantly highlighted during acute clinical situations where dynamic changes in personnel occur frequently. The Joint Commission® lists communication error among the most common causality related to sentinel events [140]. Several barriers can compromise effective communication within the medical system, including behavioral, cognitive, linguistic, environmental, and technological sources. Identifying and analyzing communication obstacles can allow for implementation of specific evidence-based solutions [134, 141].

Failures in communication and teamwork are contributors to many adverse events. For the past 10 years, emphasis has been given to team training and multiple strategies have been described [142]. Desirable teamwork behaviors include situational monitoring, communication, leadership, mutual respect, trust, role participation, and shared mental models [143]. Effective response in interdisciplinary and interprofessional collaboration is enhanced during team training. Several training programs have been created including crew resource management (CRM), which originated from the aviation industry, medical team training (MTT) at the Veteran's Health Hospitals, and the Team Strategies and Tools to Enhance Performance and Patient Safety (TeamSTEPPS) from the AHRQ. A 2020 systematic review supported the effectiveness of team training in knowledge, skills, and attitudes (KSAs) after 30 days of training [144]. This systematic review collectively described improved patient outcomes, enhanced communication, and handoff tool implementation. It has been recommended to include team-training concepts throughout the career development of all healthcare professionals [142].

8.1 Interprofessional collaboration

To optimize the patient's journey in the ICU, genuine integration of multidisciplinary coordination must be the new norm. Given the fast-paced performance pressures applied to allied health personnel (pharmacists, RT, Nutrition support, OT, PT), their current roles will evolve to participant-consultant experts for the entire unit [54].

Teaming on the fly is progressively common in critical care, especially when patients are experiencing hemodynamic instability and require emergent mechanical support. Extracorporeal membrane oxygenation can be used as a lifesaving strategy [145]. By default, this intervention requires a remarkably elevated level of interprofessional collaboration between perfusionists, respiratory therapists, physicians, physical therapists, and nurses, among many other roles.

8.2 Collective intelligence

The critical care environment is non-linear, complex, and characterized by stable and unstable equilibria. Operating as an adaptive system requires agility and a deep understanding of our interdependencies. As a result, we rely on each other's expertise to deliver the best and safest care during these critical moments of our patient's lives [146].

Every patient in the ICU is likely to benefit from the focused attention of multiple disciplines [54]. For this model to succeed, it will be essential to leverage synchronous and asynchronous communication technologies to elevate the collective intelligence. This construct is more critical than ever as we navigate diverse disciplines, engage experts from various backgrounds and generations, and integrate numerous technology-based solutions to augment the decision-making process. An example of this approach includes bedside rounds. In this activity, multiple disciplines organize daily to discuss the patient's condition, utilize various technologies such as the EMR and dashboards, and co-create the care plan.

Healthcare is moving away from the reductionist undertakings of individual performance to collective intelligence, improving the patient safety journey. We propose that there should be a deliberate institutional framework that maximizes collective intelligence, coordinating between quality improvement, patient safety, and risk management utilizing culture of safety principles to predict, prevent, and manage harm (**Figure 2**) [147].

8.3 Checklists and the checklist for early recognition and treatment of acute illness (CERTAIN) project

Checklists have been recommended as decision support tools to decrease the number of cognitive errors [148] and to encourage reflective practice [79] and metacognition [149]. Using checklists within the acute care setting and the surgical suite has led to discovering latent threats to patient safety. Medical crisis checklists have been tested in a simulated environment, demonstrating improved management during a critical medical emergency [150].

CERTAIN has been implemented across more than 55 hospitals worldwide (https://www.icertain.org/partners). Physicians, nurses, and other allied health staff from these institutions use bedside decision support tools and web-based remote simulation and coaching. Utilizing quality improvement methodology, CERTAIN implementation has demonstrated feasibility and better adherence to critical care processes in a timely manner while decreasing complications, decreasing ICU LOS, decreasing hospital LOS, and lowering mortality [151]. Another advantage of CERTAIN is the ability to provide tele-education and coaching that leads to improved costs while also improving care and outcomes in resource-limited ICUs [152].

8.4 Bundles of care and the ICU liberation project (ABCDEF)

Healthcare has shifted from the concept of caring for a critically ill patient from "ICU resuscitation and prolonged ICU stay" to an "ICU liberation" approach. The patient's outcome after an ICU stay has become a significant area of investigation, still requiring further understanding. In 2013, the Society of Critical Care Medicine and the American College of Critical Care Medicine joined forces to update the Clinical Practice Guidelines for the Management of Pain, Agitation, and Delirium in the ICU adult (ICU PAD Guidelines) published in Critical Care Medicine [153], and soon after adopted the ABDCEF Bundle of Care for the ICU setting. This bundle includes: Assess, prevent, and manage pain; B consists of both spontaneous breathing trials and spontaneous awakening trials (SAT); Choice of analgesia and sedation; Delirium: Assess, prevent, and manage; Early mobility and exercise; and Family engagement and empowerment [154] and has been named the ICU Liberation ABCDEF Bundle.

In 2018, the implementation of the ABCDEF bundle of care in 68 adult hospitals resulted in decreased mechanical ventilation days, hospital deaths, incidence of delirium, and ICU readmissions. Collectively, using all the elements of this bundle, led to a significant dose-related improvement in the outcomes measured [155]. It is noteworthy that despite these improvements, ICU providers encounter challenges implementing all the elements of the bundle reliably and consistently [156] and questions remain unanswered, which will lead to further research [157].

9. Conclusion

The initial enthusiasm to address and nullify adverse events in the health care system has clashed with the reality of a complex and ever-changing medical system prone to adverse events and medical errors. Fortunately, by approaching these complexities with the same mindset we approach complex ICU patients, we better understand the type and complexity of adverse events in medicine. This perspective has allowed the ICU community to refocus energy on quality improvement activities.

There will always be a potential for an adverse event in the intensive care practice. This understanding guides our efforts to re-engineer the healthcare delivery system in a way that minimizes risk and creates continuous learning loops for every near miss and medical error. In this review, we have proposed evidence-based mitigation strategies and solutions to develop a more robust safety culture, increase psychological safety, and encourage a more humble and inclusive leadership (**Figure 4**).

Innovation strategies with more intelligent alerts that leverage AI, and decision support tools that maximize the utility of ergonomics, human engineering, and cognitive thinking, are becoming routine. These tools will prepare the medical system to promptly recognize, triage, and intervene in high-risk situations, minimizing harm. Anticipation is a crucial element of preparation. Creating dashboards and feedback loops allow intensive care teams to respond better when facing similar clinical situations.

Most importantly, there must be an investment in the human element beyond appropriate staffing-to-acuity levels. Over and above, constant investment is needed to support the workforce using an impactful onboarding experience, a series of challenging simulation scenarios, relevant debriefing routines, stimulating professional development curricula, and promoting team dynamics. The patients and their

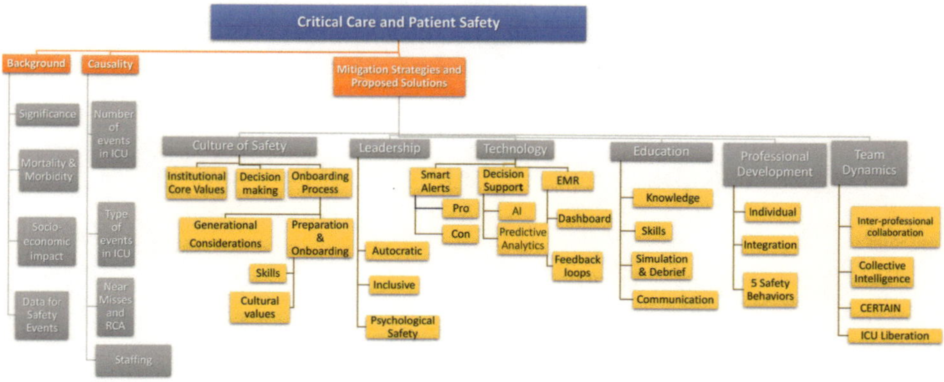

Figure 4.
Understanding risks, focusing on improvement and testing evidence based mitigation strategies and solutions. Mind-map describing how to achieve better understanding of the variables affecting safety in a patient's journey through the ICU. We also describe evidence-based mitigation strategies and possible solutions when looking at the ICU from a broader perspective including cultural aspects, leadership styles, and technological solutions. Description of retention strategies based on impactful education, stimulating professional development, and promoting team dynamics celebrating interprofessional collaboration and collective intelligence as described within the text. (Arteaga, Bacu, Moreno Franco 2022).

families are becoming an integral part of the ICU team. Together, patient safety in the ICU is fast moving towards integration and futuristic models of care.

Acknowledgements

Support from our institution, the Mayo Clinic, made possible the content and publication of this chapter. It is the Mayo Clinic's shared goal and vision that inspired the content in this chapter.

Conflict of interest

The authors declare no conflict of interest.

Notes/thanks/other declarations

We want to thank our mentors, colleagues, and learners who planted the curiosity and the desire to seek ways to improve our current medical system. Most importantly, we are grateful to our patients from whom we have learnt how to become better health care professionals and best serve their needs. Without this collaboration, the content of this chapter would have been incomplete.

Author details

Grace M. Arteaga[1*], Lilia Bacu[2] and Pablo Moreno Franco[3]

1 Mayo Clinic Rochester, Rochester, Minnesota, USA

2 Massachusetts General Hospital, Boston, Massachusetts, USA

3 Mayo Clinic Jacksonville, Jacksonville, Florida, USA

*Address all correspondence to: arteaga.grace@mayo.edu

References

[1] Dunstan E, Cook JL, Coyer F. Safety culture in intensive care internationally and in Australia: A narrative review of the literature. Australian Critical Care. 2019;**32**(6):524-539. DOI: 10.1016/j.aucc.2018.11.003

[2] Vincent CA. Research into medical accidents: A case of negligence? BMJ. 1989;**299**(6708):1150-1153. DOI: 10.1136/bmj.299.6708.1150

[3] Brennan TA et al. Incidence of adverse events and negligence in hospitalized patients. Results of the Harvard medical practice study I. The New England Journal of Medicine. 1991;**324**(6):370-376. DOI: 10.1056/NEJM199102073240604

[4] Institute of Medicine (US) Committee on Quality of Health Care in America. In: Kohn LT, Corrigan JM, Donaldson MS, editors. To Err is Human: Building a Safer Health System. Washington, DC, USA: National Academies Press (US); 2000. DOI: 10.17226/9728

[5] Carney M et al. The depiction of medical errors in a sample of medical television shows. Cureus. 2020;**12**(12):e11994. DOI: 10.7759/cureus.11994

[6] Millenson ML. Pushing the profession: How the news media turned patient safety into a priority. Quality & Safety in Health Care. 2002;**11**(1):57-63. DOI: 10.1136/qhc.11.1.57

[7] Li JW et al. Perceptions of medical errors in cancer care: An analysis of how the news media describe sentinel events. Journal of Patient Safety. 2015;**11**(1):42-51. DOI: 10.1097/PTS.0000000000000039

[8] Valentin A et al. Patient safety in intensive care: Results from the multinational sentinel events evaluation (SEE) study. Intensive Care Medicine. 2006;**32**(10):1591-1598. DOI: 10.1007/s00134-006-0290-7

[9] Bracco D et al. Human errors in a multidisciplinary intensive care unit: A 1-year prospective study. Intensive Care Medicine. 2001;**27**(1):137-145. DOI: 10.1007/s001340000751

[10] Agency for Healthcare Research and Quality. Patient Safety Network Glossary. AHRQ; 2022. Available from: https://psnet.ahrq.gov/glossary-0?f%5B0%5D=glossary_az_content_title%3AE [Accessed: October 9, 2022]

[11] Makary MA, Daniel M. Medical error-the third leading cause of death in the US. BMJ. 2016;**353**:i2139. DOI: 10.1136/bmj.i2139

[12] Gaw M, Rosinia F, Diller T. Quality and the health system: Becoming a high reliability organization. Anesthesiology Clinics. 2018;**36**(2):217-226. DOI: 10.1016/j.anclin.2018.01.010

[13] Levinson DR. Adverse Events In Hospitals: National Incidence Among Medicare Beneficiaries. Washington, DC: Department of Health and Human Services, Office of the Inspector General; 2010. p. 81

[14] Grimm CA. Adverse Events in Hospitals: a Quarter of Medicare Patients Experienced Harm in October 2018. Office of Inspector General, I. General, 2022, U.S. Department of Health and Human Services: Washington, DC; p. 117

[15] Donchin O, Francis JT, Shadmehr R. Quantifying generalization

from trial-by-trial behavior of adaptive systems that learn with basis functions: Theory and experiments in human motor control. The Journal of Neuroscience. 2003;**23**(27):9032-9045

[16] Andrews LB et al. An alternative strategy for studying adverse events in medical care. Lancet. 1997;**349**(9048):309-313. DOI: 10.1016/S0140-6736(96)08268-2

[17] Alghamdi AA et al. Prevalence and nature of medication errors and preventable adverse drug events in paediatric and neonatal intensive care settings: A systematic review. Drug Safety. 2019;**42**(12):1423-1436. DOI: 10.1007/s40264-019-00856-9

[18] Cullen DJ et al. Preventable adverse drug events in hospitalized patients: A comparative study of intensive care and general care units. Critical Care Medicine. 1997;**25**(8):1289-1297. DOI:10.1097/00003246-199708000-00014

[19] Rothschild JM et al. The critical care safety study: The incidence and nature of adverse events and serious medical errors in intensive care. Critical Care Medicine. 2005;**33**(8):1694-1700. DOI: 10.1097/01.ccm.0000171609.91035.bd

[20] Donchin Y et al. A look into the nature and causes of human errors in the intensive care unit. Critical Care Medicine. 1995;**23**(2):294-300. DOI:10.1097/00003246-199502000-00015

[21] Ahmed AH et al. Outcome of adverse events and medical errors in the intensive care unit: A systematic review and meta-analysis. American Journal of Medical Quality. 2015;**30**(1):23-30. DOI: 10.1177/1062860613514770

[22] Garrouste-Orgeas M et al. Selected medical errors in the intensive care unit: Results of the IATROREF study: Parts I and II. American Journal of Respiratory and Critical Care Medicine. 2010;**181**(2):134-142. DOI: 10.1164/rccm.200812-1820OC

[23] Wong IC et al. Incidence and nature of dosing errors in paediatric medications: A systematic review. Drug Safety. 2004;**27**(9):661-670. DOI: 10.2165/00002018-200427090-00004

[24] Sutherland A, Ashcroft DM, Phipps DL. Exploring the human factors of prescribing errors in paediatric intensive care units. Archives of Disease in Childhood. 2019;**104**(6):588-595. DOI: 10.1136/archdischild-2018-315981

[25] DH Department of Health. An Organization with a Memory: Report of an Expert Group on Learning from Adverse Events in the NHS Chaired by the Chief Medical Officer. AHRQ; 2005. Available from: https://webarchive.nationalarchives.gov.uk/ukgwa/20130107105354/http://dh.gov.uk/prod_consum_dh/groups/dh_digitalassets/@dh/@en/documents/digitalasset/dh_4065086.pdf

[26] Noble DJ, Pronovost PJ. Underreporting of patient safety incidents reduces health care's ability to quantify and accurately measure harm reduction. Journal of Patient Safety. 2010;**6**(4):247-250. DOI: 10.1097/pts.0b013e3181fd1697

[27] Archer S et al. Development of a theoretical framework of factors affecting patient safety incident reporting: A theoretical review of the literature. BMJ Open. 2017;7(12):e017155. DOI: 10.1136/bmjopen-2017-017155

[28] Frey B, Schwappach D. Critical incident monitoring in paediatric and adult critical care: From reporting to improved patient outcomes?

Current Opinion in Critical Care. 2010;**16**(6):649-653. DOI: 10.1097/MCC.0b013e32834044d8

[29] Agency for Healthcare Research and Quality. Quality Indicator User Guide: Inpatient Quality Indicators (IQI) Composite Measures. AHRQ Quality Indicators TM U.S. Department of Health and Human Services; 2022. Available from: https://qualityindicators.ahrq.gov/

[30] Griffin FA, Resar RK. IHI global trigger tool for measuring adverse events. In: IHI Innovation Series White Paper. 2nd ed. Cambridge, MA: I.f.H. Improvement; 2009. Available from: www.IHI.org

[31] Bottle A, Jarman B, Aylin P. Hospital standardized mortality ratios: Sensitivity analyses on the impact of coding. Health Services Research. 2011;**46**(6pt1):1741-1761. DOI: 10.1111/j.1475-6773.2011.01295.x

[32] Jain M et al. Decline in ICU adverse events, nosocomial infections and cost through a quality improvement initiative focusing on teamwork and culture change. Quality & Safety in Health Care. 2006;**15**(4):235-239. DOI: 10.1136/qshc.2005.016576

[33] Devlin JW et al. Executive summary: Clinical practice guidelines for the prevention and management of Pain, agitation/sedation, delirium, immobility, and sleep disruption in adult patients in the ICU. Critical Care Medicine. 2018;**46**(9):1532-1548. DOI: 10.1097/CCM.0000000000003259

[34] Smith HAB et al. 2022 Society of critical care medicine clinical practice guidelines on prevention and management of pain, agitation, neuromuscular blockade, and delirium in critically ill pediatric patients with consideration of the ICU environment and early mobility. Pediatric Critical Care Medicine. 2022;**23**(2):e74-e110. DOI: 10.1097/PCC.0000000000002873

[35] Hsieh SJ et al. Staged implementation of awakening and breathing, coordination, delirium monitoring and management, and early mobilization bundle improves patient outcomes and reduces hospital costs. Critical Care Medicine. 2019;**47**(7):885-893. DOI: 10.1097/CCM.0000000000003765

[36] Hopkins RO et al. Two-year cognitive, emotional, and quality-of-life outcomes in acute respiratory distress syndrome. American Journal of Respiratory and Critical Care Medicine. 2005;**171**(4):340-347. DOI: 10.1164/rccm.200406-763OC

[37] Pandharipande PP et al. Long-term cognitive impairment after critical illness. The New England Journal of Medicine. 2013;**369**(14):1306-1316. DOI: 10.1056/NEJMoa1301372

[38] Needham DM et al. Improving long-term outcomes after discharge from intensive care unit: Report from a stakeholders' conference. Critical Care Medicine. 2012;**40**(2):502-509. DOI: 10.1097/CCM.0b013e318232da75

[39] Manning JC et al. Conceptualizing post intensive care syndrome in children-the PICS-p framework. Pediatric Critical Care Medicine. 2018;**19**(4):298-300. DOI: 10.1097/PCC.0000000000001476

[40] Hopkins RO, Girard TD. Medical and economic implications of cognitive and psychiatric disability of survivorship. Seminars in Respiratory and Critical Care Medicine. 2012;**33**(4):348-356. DOI: 10.1055/s-0032-1321984

[41] Iwashyna TJ. Survivorship will be the defining challenge of critical care in the 21st century. Annals of

Internal Medicine. 2010;**153**(3):204-205. DOI: 10.7326/0003-4819-153-3-201008030-00013

[42] Vogus TJ et al. Adverse events and burnout: The moderating effects of workgroup identification and safety climate. Medical Care. 2020;**58**(7):594-600. DOI: 10.1097/MLR.0000000000001341

[43] Winning AM et al. The emotional impact of errors or adverse events on healthcare providers in the NICU: The protective role of coworker support. Journal of Advanced Nursing. 2018;**74**(1):172-180. DOI: 10.1111/jan.13403

[44] Scott SD et al. The natural history of recovery for the healthcare provider "second victim" after adverse patient events. Quality & Safety in Health Care. 2009;**18**(5):325-330. DOI: 10.1136/qshc.2009.032870

[45] Latif A et al. National study on the distribution, causes, and consequences of voluntarily reported medication errors between the ICU and non-ICU settings. Critical Care Medicine. 2013;**41**(2):389-398. DOI: 10.1097/CCM.0b013e318274156a

[46] Kaur AP et al. The impact of errors on healthcare professionals in the critical care setting. Journal of Critical Care. 2019;**52**:16-21. DOI: 10.1016/j.jcrc.2019.03.001

[47] Institute for Healthcare Improvement. Free from Harm: Accelerating Patient Safety Improvement Fifteen Years after To Err Is Human. Executive Summary. National Patient Safety Foundation IHI; 2015. Available from: https://www.ihi.org/resources/Pages/Publications/Free-from-Harm-Accelerating-Patient-Safety-Improvement.aspx [Accessed: 09 June 2022]

[48] Donabedian A. The quality of care. How can it be assessed? JAMA. 1988;**260**(12):1743-1748. DOI: 10.1001/jama.260.12.1743

[49] Layde PM et al. Patient safety efforts should focus on medical injuries. JAMA. 2002;**287**(15):1993-1997. DOI: 10.1001/jama.287.15.1993

[50] Lambert BL et al. The "seven pillars" response to patient safety incidents: Effects on medical liability processes and outcomes. Health Services Research. 2016;**51**(Suppl. 3):2491-2515. DOI: 10.1111/1475-6773.12548

[51] Edelson DP et al. Improving in-hospital cardiac arrest process and outcomes with performance debriefing. Archives of Internal Medicine. 2008;**168**(10):1063-1069. DOI: 10.1001/archinte.168.10.1063

[52] Patterson PD et al. Emergency healthcare worker sleep, fatigue, and alertness behavior survey (SFAB): Development and content validation of a survey tool. Accident; Analysis and Prevention. 2014;**73**:399-411. DOI: 10.1016/j.aap.2014.09.028

[53] Paterson C et al. The safe day call: Reducing silos in health care through frontline risk assessment. Joint Commission Journal on Quality and Patient Safety. 2014;**40**(10):476-471. DOI: 10.1016/s1553-7250(14)40061-8

[54] Donovan AL et al. Interprofessional care and teamwork in the ICU. Critical Care Medicine. 2018;**46**(6):980-990. DOI: 10.1097/CCM.0000000000003067

[55] Ervin JN et al. Teamwork in the intensive care unit. The American Psychologist. 2018;**73**(4):468-477. DOI: 10.1037/amp0000247

[56] Chamberlain-Salaun J, Mills J, Usher K. Terminology used to describe

health care teams: An integrative review of the literature. Journal of Multidisciplinary Healthcare. 2013;**6**: 65-74. DOI: 10.2147/JMDH.S40676

[57] Alexanian JA et al. Beyond the team: Understanding interprofessional work in two North American ICUs. Critical Care Medicine. 2015;**43**(9):1880-1886. DOI: 10.1097/CCM.0000000000001136

[58] Soltys F et al. The importance of shared decision-making in the neonatal intensive care unit. Journal of Perinatology. 2020;**40**(3):504-509. DOI: 10.1038/s41372-019-0507-6

[59] Weber U et al. Predictors of family dissatisfaction with support during neurocritical care shared decision-making. Neurocritical Care. 2021;**35**(3):714-722. DOI: 10.1007/s12028-021-01211-6

[60] Barwise A et al. Navigating the stages of and contributors to diagnostic error and delay. In: Society of Critical Care Medicine Annual Conference, Research Snapshot Theater: Quality and Patient Safety VII. Society of Critical Care Medicine and Wolters Kluwer Health Inc; 2020. p. 656. DOI: 10.1097/01.ccm.0000645348.42102.b1

[61] Cifra CL et al. Diagnostic errors in Pediatric critical care: A systematic review. Pediatric Critical Care Medicine. 2021;**22**(8):701-712. DOI: 10.1097/PCC.0000000000002735

[62] Raffel KE et al. Prevalence and characterisation of diagnostic error among 7-day all-cause hospital medicine readmissions: A retrospective cohort study. BMJ Quality and Safety. 2020;**29**(12):971-979. DOI: 10.1136/bmjqs-2020-010896

[63] Custer JW et al. Diagnostic errors in the pediatric and neonatal ICU: A systematic review. Pediatric Critical Care Medicine. 2015;**16**(1):29-36. DOI: 10.1097/PCC.0000000000000274

[64] The Leapfrog Group. When hospitals and surgery centers say "I'm sorry". The Leapfrog Group; 2006. Available from: https://www.leapfroggroup.org/influencing/never-events [Accessed: October 9, 2022]

[65] Lembitz A, Clarke TJ. Clarifying "never events" and introducing "always events". Patient Safety in Surgery. 2009;**3**:26. DOI: 10.1186/1754-9493-3-26

[66] National Coordinating Council for Medication Error Reporting and Prevention. NCC MERP Index for Categorizing Medication Errors. National Coordinating Council for Medication Error Reporting and Prevention. 2022. Available from: https://www.nccmerp.org/sites/default/files/index-color-2021-draft-change-10-2022.pdf [Accessed: August 7, 2022]

[67] Vincent C. Understanding and responding to adverse events. The New England Journal of Medicine. 2003;**348**(11):1051-1056. DOI: 10.1056/NEJMhpr020760

[68] Reason J. The contribution of latent human failures to the breakdown of complex systems. Philosophical Transactions of the Royal Society of London. Series B, Biological Sciences. 1990;**327**(1241):475-484. DOI: 10.1098/rstb.1990.0090

[69] Jung OS et al. Resilience vs. vulnerability: Psychological safety and reporting of near misses with varying proximity to harm in radiation oncology. Joint Commission Journal on Quality and Patient Safety. 2020;**47**(1):15-22. DOI: 10.1016/j.jcjq.2020.09.005

[70] Gray BM et al. Changes in stress and workplace shortages reported by U.S. critical care physicians

treating coronavirus disease 2019 patients. Critical Care Medicine. 2021;**49**(7):1068-1082. DOI: 10.1097/CCM.0000000000004974

[71] Kumaraiah DYN, Ivascu N, Hill L. Innovative ICU physician care models: Covid-19 pandemic at New York-presbyterian. NEJM Catalyst. 28 Apr 2020;**4**:2-5. DOI: 10.1056/CAT.20.0158

[72] Meissen H et al. The future of critical care: Optimizing technologies and a learning healthcare system to potentiate a more humanistic approach to critical care. Critical Care Explorations. 2022;**4**(3):e0659. DOI: 10.1097/CCE.0000000000000659

[73] Lasater KB et al. Chronic hospital nurse understaffing meets COVID-19: An observational study. BMJ Quality and Safety. 2021;**30**(8):639-647. DOI: 10.1136/bmjqs-2020-011512

[74] Almenyan AA, Albuduh A, Al-Abbas F. Effect of nursing workload in intensive care units. Cureus. 2021;**13**(1):e12674. DOI: 10.7759/cureus.12674

[75] Berlin G, Lapointe M, Murphy M. Assessing the lingering impact of COVID-19 on the nursing workforce. In: Healthcare Systems & Services. Chicago IL, USA: McKinsey & Company; 2022. Available from: https://www.mckinsey.com/industries/healthcare-systems-and-services/our-insights/assessing-the-lingering-impact-of-covid-19-on-the-nursing-workforce [Accessed: August 11, 2022]

[76] Saintsing D, Gibson LM, Pennington AW. The novice nurse and clinical decision-making: How to avoid errors. Journal of Nursing Management. 2011;**19**(3):354-359. DOI: 10.1111/j.1365-2834.2011.01248.x

[77] Asghar R. What Millennials Want In The Workplace (And Why You Should Start Giving It To Them). Jersey City, NJ, USA: Leadership Strategy Forbes, 2014; 31 Jul 2022. Available from: https://www.forbes.com/sites/robasghar/2014/01/13/what-millennials-want-in-the-workplace-and-why-you-should-start-giving-it-to-them/?sh=7b252b2c4c40 [Accessed: August 7, 2022]

[78] Hall-Jones J et al. Onboarding employees through shared values. Journal of Research, Assessment, and Practice in Higher Education. 2018;**3**(1):1-5

[79] Mamede S, Schmidt HG, Rikers R. Diagnostic errors and reflective practice in medicine. Journal of Evaluation in Clinical Practice. 2007;**13**(1):138-145. DOI: 10.1111/j.1365-2753.2006.00638.x

[80] Norman GR et al. The causes of errors in clinical reasoning: Cognitive biases, knowledge deficits, and dual process thinking. Academic Medicine. 2017;**92**(1):23-30. DOI: 10.1097/ACM.0000000000001421

[81] Committee on Diagnositc Error in Health Care National Academies of Sciences, E., and Medicine, National Academies of Sciences, Engineering, and Medicine. In: Balogh EP, Miller BT, Ball JR, editors. Improving Diagnosis in Health Care. Washington, DC, USA: The National Academies Press; 2015. p. 472. DOI: 10.17226/21794

[82] Kahneman D. Thinking, Fast and Slow. 1st ed. New York, USA: Farrar, Straus and Giroux; 2011. pp. 24-30

[83] Stiegler MP, Tung A. Cognitive processes in anesthesiology decision making. Anesthesiology. 2014;**120**(1):204-217. DOI: 10.1097/ALN.0000000000000073

[84] Croskerry P. From mindless to mindful practice—Cognitive bias and clinical decision making. The

New England Journal of Medicine. 2013;**368**(26):2445-2448. DOI: 10.1056/NEJMp1303712

[85] Royce CS, Hayes MM, Schwartzstein RM. Teaching critical thinking: A case for instruction in cognitive biases to reduce diagnostic errors and improve patient safety. Academic Medicine. 2019;**94**(2):187-194. DOI: 10.1097/ACM.0000000000002518

[86] Hayes MM, Chatterjee S, Schwartzstein RM. Critical thinking in critical care: Five strategies to improve teaching and learning in the intensive care unit. Annals of the American Thoracic Society. 2017;**14**(4):569-575. DOI: 10.1513/AnnalsATS.201612-1009AS

[87] Owens BP, Johnson M, and Mitchell TR. Expressed humility in organization: Implications for performance, teams, and leadership. Organization Science. 2013;**24**(5):1517-1538. DOI: 10.1287/orsc.1120.0795

[88] Bourke J, Titus A. The key to inclusive leadership. In: Diversity and Inclusion. Cambridge, MA: Harvard Business Review; 2020

[89] Stoller J, Mohta NS. Leading in a VUCA World: Volatile, Uncertain, Ambiguous. NEJM Catalyst Innovations in Care Delivery. Massachusetts Medical Society [Audio] 2017. Posted August 16, 2017. Available from: https://catalyst.nejm.org/doi/full/10.1056/CAT.17.0408

[90] Curry LA et al. Influencing organisational culture to improve hospital performance in care of patients with acute myocardial infarction: A mixed-methods intervention study. BMJ Quality and Safety. 2018;**27**(3):207-217. DOI: 10.1136/bmjqs-2017-006989

[91] Nembhard IM, Edmondson AC. Making it safe: The effects of leader inclusiveness and professional status on psychological safety and improvement efforts in health care teams. Journal of Organizational Behavior. 2006;**27**:941-966. DOI: 10.1002/job.413

[92] Kim SR et al. Relationship among symptoms, resilience, post-traumatic growth, and quality of life in patients with glioma. European Journal of Oncology Nursing. 2020;**48**:101830. DOI: 10.1016/j.ejon.2020.101830

[93] Ferrere A et al. Fostering ethical conduct through psychological safety. Magazine. 2022. Available from: https://sloanreview.mit.edu/article/fostering-ethical-conduct-through-psychological-safety/ [Accessed: 08 October 2022]

[94] Edmonson A. Psychological safety and learning behavior in work teams. Administrative Science Quarterly. 1999;**44**(2):350-383. DOI: 10.2307/2666999

[95] Roloff KS, Edmonson A. Leveraging diversity through psychological safety. In: Burke S, Salas E, Goodwin GF, editors. Team Effectiveness in Complex Organizations: Cross-disciplinary Perspectives and Approaches. 1st ed. New York, USA: Routledge; 2008. p. 624

[96] Liu CE et al. Supervision incivility and employee psychological safety in the workplace. International Journal of Environmental Research and Public Health. 2020;**17**(3):840. DOI: 10.3390/ijerph17030840

[97] Baer M, Frese M. Innovation is not enough: Climates for initiative and psychological safety, process innovations, and firm performance. Journal of Organizational Behavior. 2003;**24**(1):45-68. DOI: 10.1002/job.179

[98] Hebles M, Trincado-Munoz F, Ortega K. Stress and turnover intentions

within healthcare teams: The mediating role of psychological safety, and the moderating effect of COVID-19 worry and supervisor support. Frontiers in Psychology. 2021;**12**:758438. DOI: 10.3389/fpsyg.2021.758438

[99] Coutifaris CGV, Grant AM. Taking your team behind the curtain: The effects of leader feedback-sharing and feedback-seeking on team psychological safety. Organization Science. (Catonsville, MD USA). 2021;**33**(4):1251-1699. DOI: 10.1287/orsc.2021.1498

[100] Dziadzko MA et al. Testing modes of computerized sepsis alert notification delivery systems. BMC Medical Informatics and Decision Making. 2016;**16**(1):156. DOI: 10.1186/s12911-016-0396-y

[101] Dziadzko MA et al. User perception and experience of the introduction of a novel critical care patient viewer in the ICU setting. International Journal of Medical Informatics. 2016;**88**:86-91. DOI: 10.1016/j.ijmedinf.2016.01.011

[102] Pannu SR et al. Development and validation of severe hypoxemia associated risk prediction model in 1,000 mechanically ventilated patients. Critical Care Medicine. 2015;**43**(2):308-317. DOI: 10.1097/CCM.0000000000000671

[103] Grek A et al. Sepsis and shock response team: Impact of a multidisciplinary approach to implementing surviving Sepsis campaign guidelines and surviving the process. American Journal of Medical Quality. 2017;**32**(5):500-507. DOI: 10.1177/1062860616676887

[104] Aakre C et al. Prospective validation of a near real-time EHR-integrated automated SOFA score calculator. International Journal of Medical Informatics. 2017;**103**:1-6. DOI: 10.1016/j.ijmedinf.2017.04.001

[105] Nolan ME et al. Health IT usability focus section: Data use and navigation patterns among medical ICU clinicians during electronic chart review. Applied Clinical Informatics. 2017;**8**(4):1117-1126. DOI: 10.4338/ACI-2017-06-RA-0110

[106] Cubro H et al. Cost effectiveness of intensive care in a low resource setting: A prospective cohort of medical critically ill patients. World Journal of Critical Care Medicine. 2016;**5**(2):150-164. DOI: 10.5492/wjccm.v5.i2.150

[107] Harrison AM et al. Comparison of methods of alert acknowledgement by critical care clinicians in the ICU setting. PeerJ. 2017;**5**:e3083. DOI: 10.7717/peerj.3083

[108] Pickering BW et al. Novel representation of clinical information in the ICU: Developing user interfaces which reduce information overload. Applied Clinical Informatics. 2010;**1**(2):116-131. DOI: 10.4338/ACI-2009-12-CR-0027

[109] Pickering BW et al. Clinical review: The hospital of the future - building intelligent environments to facilitate safe and effective acute care delivery. Critical Care. 2012;**16**(2):220. DOI: 10.1186/cc11142

[110] Gutierrez G. Artificial intelligence in the intensive care unit. Critical Care. 2020;**24**(1):101. DOI: 10.1186/s13054-020-2785-y

[111] Mathur P, Burns ML. Artificial Intelligence in Critical Care. International Anesthesiology Clinics. 2019;**57**(2):89-102. DOI: 10.1097/AIA.0000000000000221

[112] Cerrato P, Halamka J, Pencina M. A proposal for developing a platform that evaluates algorithmic equity and accuracy. BMJ Health & Care

Informatics. 2022;**29**(1):e100423. DOI: 10.1136/bmjhci-2021-100423

[113] Fliegenschmidt J et al. Artificial intelligence predicts delirium following cardiac surgery: A case study. Journal of Clinical Anesthesia. 2021;**75**:110473. DOI: 10.1016/j.jclinane.2021.110473

[114] Bates DW et al. The potential of artificial intelligence to improve patient safety: A scoping review. NPJ Digital Medicine. 2021;**4**(1):54. DOI: 10.1038/s41746-021-00423-6

[115] Goh KH et al. Artificial intelligence in sepsis early prediction and diagnosis using unstructured data in healthcare. Nature Communications. 2021;**12**(1):711. DOI: 10.1038/s41467-021-20910-4

[116] Cerrato P, Halamka J. The Digital Reconstruction of Healthcare: Transitioning from Brick and Mortar to Virtual Care. New York: Taylor & Francis Group: An Informa Business: HIMSS Publishing; 2021. p. 150. DOI: 10.1201/9781003094234

[117] Sutcliffe KM. High reliability organizations (HROs). Best Practice & Research. Clinical Anaesthesiology. 2011;**25**(2):133-144. DOI: 10.1016/j.bpa.2011.03.001

[118] Jha AK et al. Use of electronic health records in U.S. hospitals. The New England Journal of Medicine. 2009;**360**(16):1628-1638. DOI: 10.1056/NEJMsa0900592

[119] Simborg DW. Promoting electronic health record adoption. Is it the correct focus? Journal of the American Medical Informatics Association. 2008;**15**(2):127-129. DOI: 10.1197/jamia.M2573

[120] Pickering BW et al. The implementation of clinician designed, human-centered electronic medical record viewer in the intensive care unit: A pilot step-wedge cluster randomized trial. International Journal of Medical Informatics. 2015;**84**(5):299-307. DOI: 10.1016/j.ijmedinf.2015.01.017

[121] Bansal V et al. Early machine-human interface around sepsis severity identification: From diagnosis to improved management? Acta Medica Academica. 2018;**47**(1):27-38. DOI: 10.5644/ama2006-124.212

[122] Grek A, Markum M, Franco PM. Will SEP-1 Compliance Metrics Flood our System? Wolters Kluwer Health, Inc. Hagerstown MD USA. Critical Care Medicine. 2019;**47**(1):638. DOI: 10.1097/01.ccm.0000552067.40309.99

[123] Vincent C, Amalberti R. Approaches to safety: One size does not fit all. In: Safer Healthcare: Strategies for the Real World. 1st ed. Vol. 1. Springer Cham (CH): Springer Open; 2016. pp. 27-36. DOI: 10.1007/978-3-319-25559-0

[124] Motola I et al. Simulation in healthcare education: A best evidence practical guide. AMEE Guide No. 82. Medical Teacher. 2013;**35**(10):e1511-e1530. DOI: 10.3109/0142159X.2013.818632

[125] Beal MD et al. The effectiveness of medical simulation in teaching medical students critical care medicine: A systematic review and Meta-analysis. Simulation in Healthcare. 2017;**12**(2):104-116. DOI: 10.1097/SIH.0000000000000189

[126] Cook DA et al. Mastery learning for health professionals using technology-enhanced simulation: A systematic review and meta-analysis. Academic Medicine. 2013;**88**(8):1178-1186. DOI: 10.1097/ACM.0b013e31829a365d

[127] Issenberg SB et al. Features and uses of high-fidelity medical

simulations that lead to effective learning: A BEME systematic review. Medical Teacher. 2005;**27**(1):10-28. DOI: 10.1080/01421590500046924

[128] Cheng A et al. Debriefing for technology-enhanced simulation: A systematic review and meta-analysis. Medical Education. 2014;**48**(7):657-666. DOI: 10.1111/medu.12432

[129] Dieckmann P et al. Variation and adaptation: Learning from success in patient safety-oriented simulation training. Advances in Simulation (London). 2017;**2**:21. DOI: 10.1186/s41077-017-0054-1

[130] Schmidt E et al. Simulation exercises as a patient safety strategy: A systematic review. Annals of Internal Medicine. 2013;**158**(5 Pt 2):426-432. DOI: 10.7326/0003-4819-158-5-201303051-00010

[131] Colman N et al. Designing for patient safety and efficiency: Simulation-based hospital design testing. HERD. 2020;**13**(4):68-80. DOI: 10.1177/1937586720921777

[132] Grek A et al. Interviewing critical care nurse practitioners and physician assistants using a simulation center. Critical Care Medicine. 2018;**46**(1):40. DOI: 10.1097/01.ccm.0000528134.11532.65

[133] Kon AA et al. Shared decision-making in intensive care units. Executive summary of the American College of Critical Care Medicine and American Thoracic Society Policy Statement. American Journal of Respiratory and Critical Care Medicine. 2016;**193**(12):1334-1336. DOI: 10.1164/rccm.201602-0269ED

[134] Schnipper JL et al. Approach to Improving Patient Safety: Communication. PSNet Collection, Annual Perspective. Rockville. MD, USA: AHRQ; 10 Mar 2021. Available from: https://psnet.ahrq.gov/perspective/approach-improving-patient-safety-communication [Accessed: August 9, 2022]

[135] Dendere R et al. Patient portals facilitating engagement with inpatient electronic medical records: A systematic review. Journal of Medical Internet Research. 2019;**21**(4):e12779. DOI: 10.2196/12779

[136] Bosslet GT et al. An official ATS/AACN/ACCP/ESICM/SCCM policy statement: Responding to requests for potentially inappropriate treatments in intensive care units. American Journal of Respiratory and Critical Care Medicine. 2015;**191**(11):1318-1330. DOI: 10.1164/rccm.201505-0924ST

[137] Jacobowski NL et al. Communication in critical care: Family rounds in the intensive care unit. American Journal of Critical Care. 2010;**19**(5):421-430. DOI: 10.4037/ajcc2010656

[138] Heyland DK et al. Family satisfaction with care in the intensive care unit: Results of a multiple center study. Critical Care Medicine. 2002;**30**(7):1413-1418. DOI: 10.1097/00003246-200207000-00002

[139] Wall RJ et al. Family satisfaction in the ICU: Differences between families of survivors and nonsurvivors. Chest. 2007;**132**(5):1425-1433. DOI: 10.1378/chest.07-0419

[140] Joint Commission. Sentinel Event Alert 58: Inadequate Hand-off Communication. Oakbrook Terrace, IL, USA: The Joint Commission; 2017. Available from: https://www.jointcommission.org/resources/patient-safety-topics/sentinel-event/sentinel-event-alert-newsletters/

sentinel-event-alert-58-inadequate-hand-off-communication/#.YxtvCbTMKUk [Accessed: 09 September 2022]

[141] Guttman OT et al. Dissecting communication barriers in healthcare: A path to enhancing communication resiliency, reliability, and patient safety. Journal of Patient Safety. 2021;**17**(8):e1465-e1471. DOI: 10.1097/PTS.0000000000000541

[142] Weaver SJ, Dy SM, Rosen MA. Team-training in healthcare: A narrative synthesis of the literature. BMJ Quality and Safety. 2014;**23**(5):359-372. DOI: 10.1136/bmjqs-2013-001848

[143] Manser T. Teamwork and patient safety in dynamic domains of healthcare: A review of the literature. Acta Anaesthesiologica Scandinavica. 2009;**53**(2):143-151. DOI: 10.1111/j.1399-6576.2008.01717.x

[144] Costar DM, Hall KK. Improving team performance and patient safety on the job through team training and performance support tools: A systematic review. Journal of Patient Safety. 2020;**16**(3S Suppl 1):S48-S56. DOI: 10.1097/PTS.0000000000000746

[145] Sheasby J et al. An interprofessional approach to mobilizing patients with COVID-19 receiving extracorporeal membrane oxygenation. AACN Advanced Critical Care. 2022;**3**(3): 262-273. DOI: https://doi. org/10.4037/aacnacc2022293

[146] Mayo AT, Woolley AW. Teamwork in health care: Maximizing collective intelligence via inclusive collaboration and open communication. AMA Journal of Ethics. 2016;**18**(9):933-940. DOI: 10.1001/journalofethics.2016.18.9.stas2-1609

[147] Liao M, Tan N. Collective intelligence of peer learning: Promoting culture of learning and improvement among radiologists. Current Problems in Diagnostic Radiology. 2021;**50**(6):761-763. DOI: 10.1067/j.cpradiol.2020.09.017

[148] Ely JW, Graber ML, Croskerry P. Checklists to reduce diagnostic errors. Academic Medicine. 2011;**86**(3):307-313. DOI: 10.1097/ACM.0b013e31820824cd

[149] Croskerry P. The importance of cognitive errors in diagnosis and strategies to minimize them. Academic Medicine. 2003;**78**(8):775-780

[150] Dryver E et al. Medical crisis checklists in the emergency department: A simulation-based multi-institutional randomised controlled trial. BMJ Quality and Safety. 2021;**30**(9):697-705. DOI: 10.1136/bmjqs-2020-012740

[151] Vukoja M et al. Checklist for early recognition and treatment of acute illness: International collaboration to improve critical care practice. World Journal of Critical Care Medicine. 2015;**4**(1):55-61. DOI: 10.5492/wjccm.v4.i1.55

[152] Kovacevic P et al. Impact of weekly case-based tele-education on quality of care in a limited resource medical intensive care unit. Critical Care. 2019;**23**(1):220. DOI: 10.1186/s13054-019-2494-6

[153] Barr J et al. Clinical practice guidelines for the management of pain, agitation, and delirium in adult patients in the intensive care unit: Executive summary. American Journal of Health-System Pharmacy. 2013;**70**(1):53-58. DOI: 10.1093/ajhp/70.1.53

[154] Marra A et al. The ABCDEF bundle in critical care. Critical Care Clinics. 2017;**33**(2):225-243. DOI: 10.1016/j.ccc.2016.12.005

[155] Pun BT et al. Caring for critically ill patients with the ABCDEF bundle: Results of the ICU liberation collaborative in over 15,000 adults. Critical Care Medicine. 2019;**47**(1):3-14. DOI: 10.1097/CCM.0000000000003482

[156] Balas MC et al. Common challenges to effective ABCDEF bundle implementation: The ICU liberation campaign experience. Critical Care Nurse. 2019;**39**(1):46-60. DOI: 10.4037/ccn2019927

[157] Stollings JL et al. Implementing the ABCDEF bundle: Top 8 questions asked during the ICU liberation ABCDEF bundle improvement collaborative. Critical Care Nurse. 2019;**39**(1):36-45. DOI: 10.4037/ccn2019981

Chapter 8

Patient Safety in Physiotherapy: Are Errors that Cause or Could Cause Harm Preventable?

Griselda Gonzalez-Caminal, Aida Camps Gomez and Carmen Gomar-Sancho

Abstract

The concept of patient safety is less developed in physiotherapy than in other areas of health care. Standard physiotherapy care, whether active or passive, is largely viewed as harmless as it is not associated with serious adverse events. Physiotherapists, however, are increasingly involved in the care of in-hospital patients, in particular for early rehabilitation for patients who are critically ill or have undergone complex surgery. The increased risk of serious adverse events in such settings has contributed to an increased awareness of safety in physiotherapy. Most practitioners, however, operate in non-hospital settings, where the idea that physiotherapy causes little or no harm is more deeply entrenched and does little to foster a culture of risk awareness or encourage practitioners to report or record errors. Error reporting and recording are two basic pillars of patient safety and should be extended to all health care areas. Heightened awareness and the creation of systems that encourage reporting will gradually lead to the creation of a culture of safety in physiotherapy.

Keywords: physiotherapy, patient safety, adverse events, rehabilitation, errors, risk of harm

1. Introduction

Patient safety is a fundamental principle of health care derived from the Latin dictum *primum non nocere* (First do no harm) [1]. Despite common belief, this phrase was not part of the original Hippocratic Oath; it is deeply embedded in the medical profession [2, 3] and one of the pillars of the bioethical principle of nonmaleficence. Nonmaleficence, which was included in the Hippocratic Oath, is an umbrella principle under which medicine is practiced and should be applicable to all health care professions [4].

The axiom "do no harm" lies at the center of patient safety, which is defined by the World Health Organization (WHO) as "a framework of organized activities that creates cultures, processes, procedures, behaviors, technologies, and environments in health care" [5]. According to Rocco and Garrido [6], this framework represents a "conscious attempt to avoid injury to the patient caused by care [...] and is the precondition for the performance of any clinical activity."

Safety is a primary concern in any activity involving risk. Safety systems originated in the aviation and nuclear industries and were introduced into medicine in the late 1950s by anesthesia practitioners facing costly insurance plans to cover liability for damages relating to anesthesia-related complications and deaths, which were frequent at the time [7]. The push for patient safety in mainstream medicine, however, began with the publication of the 2000 landmark report "To Err is Human: Building a safer health system," which brought attention to the high rates of medical errors in the US health care [8]. This report led to studies in other countries, which revealed similar findings, prompting the creation of the WHO World Alliance for Patient Safety in 2004 and the first concerted efforts to create mechanisms and systems aimed at reducing errors and improving safety.

Unsafe care remains one of the top ten causes of death and disability worldwide, with recent data suggesting that unsafe hospital-based care causes 134 million adverse events (AEs) each year and contributes to 2.6 million annual deaths in low- and middle-income countries [9]. Berner and Graber [10], in their study of overconfidence as a cause of diagnostic error in medicine, reported that 35% of physicians surveyed stated that they or a family member had experienced a medical error in the past five years. An estimated 10–15% of health care expenditure has been directly linked to patient harm [11], which on a global scale is the equivalent of US$ 1 trillion to 2 trillion every year [9]. Similar findings have been reported in Spain [12, 13], as well as in many countries.

Early reports on safety risks in health care focused on adverse effects (AEs) results of the individual work of doctors, but they also brought to light an increasingly complex, interacting, and health care system in which AEs were caused by both doctors and other members of the health care team. The reports, however, also identified opportunities for teams to proactively work together to protect patients from preventable adverse outcomes.

As nurses work in tandem with doctors across all areas of care delivery, patient safety has steadily become an integral part of their practice. This is not the case, however, with physiotherapy. One of the reasons why patient safety is still in its early stages is the scarcity of data and resulting lack of awareness about error and safety. Combined, this impedes a culture where physiotherapists are inclined to disclose or report incidents, a practice that in medical practice has allowed their analysis and led to the implementation of preventive patient safety strategies and actions [14–17].

The objective of this chapter is to show that physiotherapy has not been integrated into the patient safety culture that is integrated into the daily activity of other branches of health sciences. The scarcity of information in the literature or the field of professional societies does not mean that physiotherapy does not have adverse effects. Lack of evidence does not mean absence, and absence does not mean evidence. The data search comes from the interest, and the interest comes from awareness of the problem. Our goal is to arouse interest in the possibility of adverse effects in physiotherapy and its study and to provide the concepts of patient safety that are applied in other professions.

2. Methods

Review chapter. Pubmed and PEDro databases were searched through June–July 2022 to identify relevant articles related to patient safety in physiotherapy field.

KEYWORDS
"physiotherapy" or "rehabilitation" AND "patient safety"
"physiotherapy" AND "malpractice"
"physiotherapy" AND "patient safety" AND "treatment effects" OR "secondary effects"
"physiotherapy" AND "intensive care unit" AND "patient safety"
"physiotherapy" AND "patient safety" OR "effects" AND "manipulation"

Table 1.
Search strategy.

All databases were searched by using the following keywords: patient safety and physiotherapy or rehabilitation combined with keywords related to physiotherapy and patient safety, such as treatment effects, malpractice, secondary effects, consequences, manipulation, and intensive care unit. The search strategy is presented in **Table 1**.

To obtain relevant articles, the search results were screened, using the following inclusion criteria: (1) the study is published after January 2007, (2) articles are published in English, Portuguese, or Spanish, and (3) the physiotherapy intervention is described in papers, where treatment is implemented. Screening for eligibility was

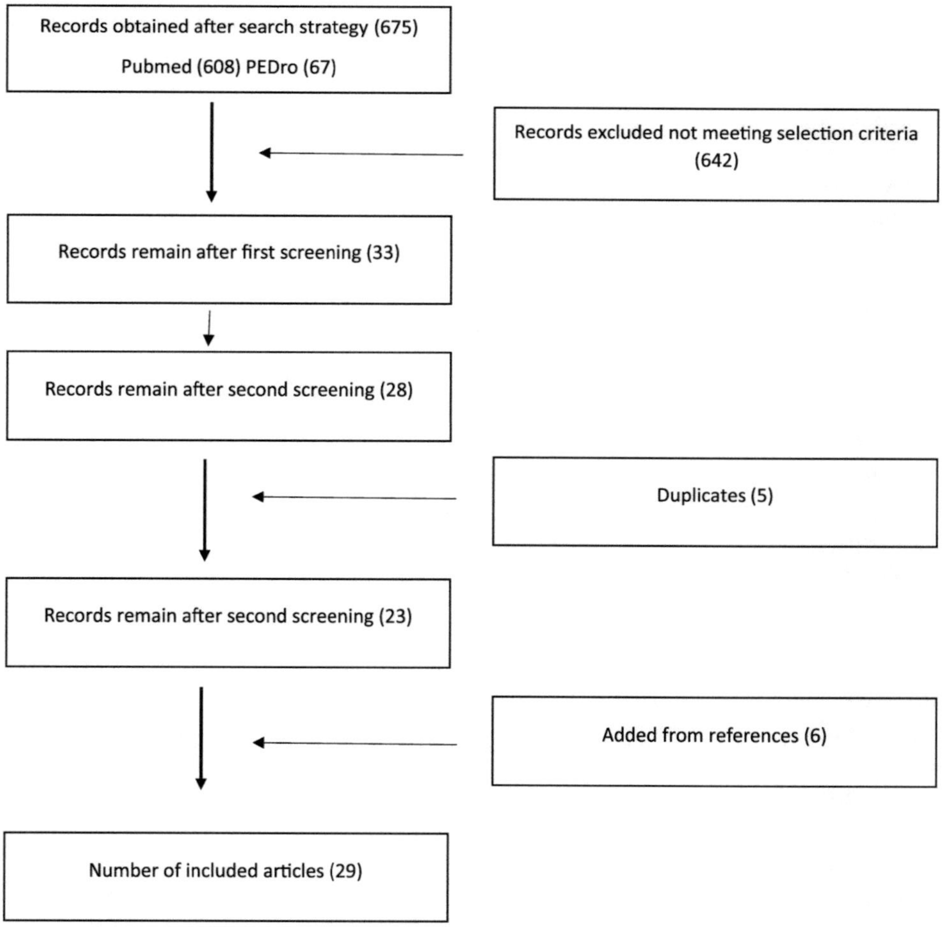

Figure 1.
Flow Chart of study selection.

first performed on title and abstract. Then, full-text versions were obtained. In the second phase, the full-text version was screened. Books and other documents were excluded. The reference lists of reviewed articles were also searched for relevant citations. Relevant literature from medical side was also included to complete general concepts in the introduction based on patient safety health care perspective. The final search provided a total of 29 studies (see **Figure 1**: flow chart of the study selection) directly related to physiotherapy. All other sources use in the paper are from other fields and or directly related to patient safety, bioethics, and malpractice as concepts and/or analyzed in a medical or other health professions.

3. Physiotherapy and patient safety

Physiotherapy is a much more recent profession than either medicine or nursing. Although it has gained widespread acceptance and is increasingly understood, greater efforts are needed to increase awareness of its function and role among the general population and other health care professionals [16, 18–20].

The World Confederation of Physical Therapy (WCPT) is the sole international voice for physiotherapists. Through national member organizations, it represents, regulates, and coordinates both profession and its practitioners, and its mission is to promote high standards of practice, education, and research [21–23]. The WCPT defines physiotherapy as services provided "to develop, maintain and restore maximum movement and functional ability throughout the lifespan", including "services in circumstances, where movement and function are threatened by aging, injury, pain, diseases, disorders, conditions, and/or environmental factors and with the understanding that functional movement is central to what it means to be healthy" [21].

The process of physiotherapy care involves the following stages: examination, evaluation, diagnosis and prognosis, intervention or treatment, re-examination, and discharge. Interventions and treatments include therapeutic exercise; functional training in self-care and home management; functional training in work, community and leisure; manual therapy (including mobilization and manipulation); prescription, application, and, as appropriate, fabrication of devices and equipment (assistive, adaptive, orthotic, protective, supportive, and prosthetic); airway clearance; integumentary repair and protection; electrotherapeutic modalities; physical agents and mechanical modalities; patient-related instruction; and coordination, communication, and documentation [21]. Services also include specialized interventions, such as intravaginal exercises for incontinence and dry needling.

Physiotherapists are autonomous practitioners who manage and treat chronic, subacute, and acute conditions. Direct access to physiotherapy (the ability to consult a regulated physiotherapist without the need for referral) is now an option in some (Australia, The Netherlands, or Canada) countries [20, 24–26]. Enormous advances have been made in professional autonomy and evidence-based practice in physiotherapy [4, 21, 27]. Nonetheless, while evidence-based practice is now widely recognized in this field, awareness of a number of basic bioethical principles that have been fully integrated into other professions, such as medicine or nursing is still lacking in physiotherapy [14, 16, 19, 28, 29].

The practice of physiotherapy involves the application of active and passive techniques, as described above. These techniques are generally viewed as harmless, as they do not result in serious AEs [22]. The perception, however, that standard physiotherapy care causes minimal or no harm favors a culture where errors are not recognized, reported, registered, or analyzed for corrective or preventive action. Physiotherapists are increasingly involved in the care of in-hospital patients, particularly intensive care patients and those requiring early rehabilitation after complex surgery [30–32]. Because work of this nature can significantly interfere with the outcomes of physiotherapeutic treatments and result in serious AEs, general awareness of patient safety is increasing in these settings [14, 17]. Like in other health care professions, errors can also occur during the application of increasingly sophisticated technologies. That said the vast majority of physiotherapists work in non-hospital settings and private practices [33]. Private practice work could be a barrier to the development of effective data collection processes and creates a reliance on internal control systems for reporting and recording incidents and notifying the pertinent authorities.

AE reporting, recording, and analysis are the pillars of patient safety systems [9] and must be implemented across all areas of health care, both in and outside hospitals and in the public and private sectors [7].

4. Critical concepts: the link between malpractice and patient safety

Data are essential for guiding the implementation of patient safety systems but are very scarce in the field of physiotherapy [17]. Information on errors and AEs in the health sciences comes from critical incident reports, complaints, malpractice or fraudulence claims, preventable death reports, and audits. While these reports contain indirect indicators of safety failures, [9, 17] they show just the tip of the iceberg. In addition, they focus on outcomes rather than processes.

A clear understanding of what constitutes an error and an AE is necessary for effective reporting and recording, and in the framework of patient safety, it is particularly important to distinguish between malpractice and error. The literature contains reports of malpractice in physiotherapy [34]. Malpractice is wrongful conduct by a health care professional that causes injury to a patient. It always involves negligence and legal responsibility [35]. Most AEs, however, are unintended and caused by human error or latent system errors missed by humans [36–38].

According to Reason's theory of human error, safety is a complex and multilayered system [39]. The basic premise is that humans are fallible and as a result, errors will occur, despite attempts to prevent them. This is why it is imperative to implement effective detection, prevention, and mitigation systems [40].

The predominant focus on assigning individual blame for AEs impeded advances in patient safety for many years, as the tendency was to cover up errors out of fear of personal consequences. In the present culture of patient safety, it is recognized that errors will occur because humans are fallible; biological systems are inherently complex (systemic alterations, for example, can occur during respiratory physiotherapy of patients with neurological disorders), and organizational and working systems have functional weak points (latent errors). The goal of patient safety is to identify weaknesses in each of the above dimensions and evaluate and decide which measures should be implemented to safeguard against what are mostly preventable errors [9, 17, 40]. As WHO has stated in several of its documents, most AEs are preventable [1, 5, 8].

In professions, such as physiotherapy, where patient safety is still in its infancy and error perception and recognition are lacking, error analyses tend to focus on individual blame rather than on the components of the process leading up to the error. These analyses thus tend to be based on a deficient understanding of the care process and an

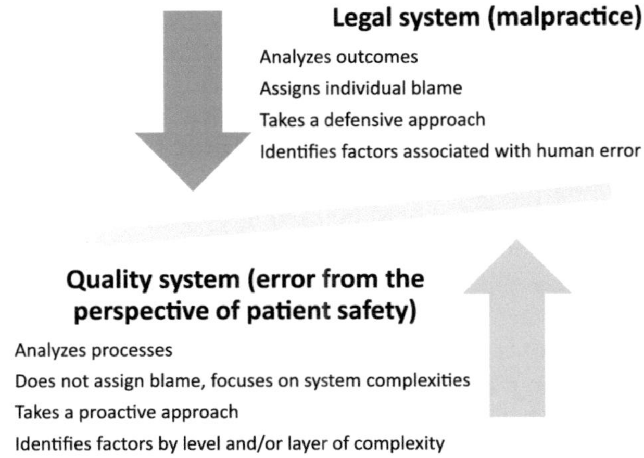

Figure 2.
Scales comparing the legal and quality systems.

excessive focus on "intentionality" (active errors). The focal point is, therefore, one malpractice, which is a criminal act that is directly or indirectly punishable [41].

Without a climate of trust in which errors are viewed as an opportunity for learning and improvement rather than a cause for blame, it is difficult to create a safety culture [9, 40]. Patient safety is not about malpractice, it is about human factors and systems, which both have their limitations. It is about detecting problems that could have been prevented and implementing the necessary steps to ensure that they do not recur [38, 42]. It is about being proactive rather than defensive, which is the typical approach in malpractice cases [43].

As stated by Di Luca et al. [36] "The healthcare disciplines of patient safety and risk management are deeply interrelated and interdependent. Patient safety alone is blind to consequences beyond outcome, and risk management alone can manage and mitigate but not prevent errors" [36]. Actions were taken to reduce the risk of malpractice, and its legislative consequences have not resulted in improved patient safety indicators [35, 38]. It is thus important to understand the differences between the two concepts. It would, however, also be interesting to analyze their interconnections, as they probably have overlapping or complementary features (**Figure 2**) [36, 37]. When faced with a malpractice claim, it is essential to conduct a root-cause analysis of what occurred from the perspective of patient safety to gain an overall picture that captures the complementary aspects of both the legal and the quality system.

Investigations into patient safety and AEs serve to minimize risks and errors in care processes and/or related administrative processes. Scheirton et al. [44] identified six types of errors and AEs in the field of occupational and physical therapy practice:

- Faulty material that results in a patient falling and is not reported
- False reporting of data and cover-up of a colleague
- Substandard care and fraud whereby a practitioner records treating a patient seen by another practitioner due to staff shortages

- Poor communication during patient handover
- Forgetting about and neglecting the needs of a patient
- Ill-treatment of a patient and cover-up of the practitioner responsible for this treatment

Other authors in the field have analyzed AEs, risk factors, and effects associated with different types of physiotherapy techniques, modalities, and situations, such as dry needling [45], manual therapy [46–51], hospital falls, and early mobilization in orthopedic [30, 32, 52] and/or intensive care patients [31].

Data collection is also useful for determining procedures and techniques, in addition to being beneficial, which are effective and safe to implement, such as mobilization and rehabilitation in intensive care units [53], active mobilization in patients requiring continuous renal replacement therapy [54], cancer rehabilitation [55], lower limb plyometric training in older adults [56], and cervical traction and exercise in patients with neck pain (clinical prediction rule to identify, which patients are most likely to benefit) [57].

Most studies of AEs in physiotherapy have focused on the intervention stage of the care process, but many techniques used for treatment are also used for diagnostic purposes (e.g., neurodynamic tests) [58, 59]. Accordingly, data collected on interventions could be extrapolated to other stages of the care pathway (e.g., evaluation). Errors that occur in later stages of the process are linked to errors or decisions made earlier on. A poor evaluation thus can lead to misdiagnosis (**Table 2**). If efficient reporting and recording systems are to be created, physiotherapists must be involved in the development of quality systems [17, 60] and have a clear understanding of the data generated.

Examination	Inappropriate facilities Insufficient time Lack of information on previous procedures (e.g., surgical approach used)
Evaluation	Inappropriate facilities Incorrect manipulation Insufficient or excessive tissue stretching Inappropriate use of material or equipment Lack of patient information due to lack of expertize (e.g., not asking for comorbidities focusing on current situation)
Diagnosis prognosis	Incorrect diagnosis
Intervention – treatment	Inappropriate facilities Incorrect manipulation Insufficient or excessive tissue stretching Inappropriate use of material or equipment
Re-Examination	Insufficient or excessive tissue stretching Inappropriate use of material or equipment
Discharge	Any error from the previous stages resulting in poor re-evaluation, inadequate treatment, or early termination of treatment

Table 2.
Errors that can occur during the different stages of physiotherapy care process.

5. Potential errors: from minor to major consequences

Most in-hospital care have a strong safety culture in which the different components and layers of patient safety are strongly embedded in both medical and nursing practice [61], probably because working in these settings carries more risks as it involves more invasive and complex techniques and procedures. In physiotherapy, by contrast, AEs are generally classified as minor (no-harm) events or near misses (incidents that do not cause harm to the patient) [42]. Examples are interference with equipment or devices during mobilization of a critically ill patient, a mild burn sustained during heat therapy, or a near fall when transferring a patient from one chair to another. Interprofessional and multiprofessional collaboration is also at a more nascent stage in physiotherapy than in medicine, where the doctor/nurse tandem is well established [61].

Although no-harm and near-miss events may be anywhere between 7 and 100 times more common than AEs, systems for reporting them are much less common [62]. These less-impactful events represent latent system risks that must be reported to prevent serious consequences in the future [63]. High incidence rates have been reported for these events in physiotherapy, but the fact that they cause few consequences has probably contributed to general perception of physiotherapy care being harmless [50].

Invasive procedures, such as dry needling, however, are becoming more common in physiotherapy and certain rehabilitation treatments with the potential to cause serious AEs (e.g., early rehabilitation of orthopedic surgery patients, respiratory and neuromuscular physiotherapy in intensive care patients, and manual treatment of spinal cord injuries) are already in wide use [32, 51]. Incorrect mobilization after prosthetic orthopedic surgery can undo the results of surgery [52], while detailed knowledge and extreme care are needed when delivering treatment to a critically ill patient whose life depends on certain machines or devices (e.g., respirators, intravascular catheters, or hemodialysis machines) [32, 53]. Patients in intensive care units or orthopedic departments after surgery require specialized and highly protocolized care. In such environments, the therapeutic development of physiotherapy will be safe as long as the patient safety culture is well established. Recommendations in those fields need to be more extensively practiced and researched to deepen the discussion.

To manage the risks associated with a given treatment, one must not only be aware that they exist but also understand their severity (see example in **Figure 3**) and potential impact. Such an awareness will favor the reporting of incidents by both physiotherapists and other agents [64].

Analyses of risk prevention should also incentivize reporting [9]. Research in physiotherapy has been increasing in recent decades. This means that more and more information is available on the effectiveness of the applied treatments. Information is also available on their risks. Creating this scientific awareness should, little by little, help to also build an awareness of patient safety, which inevitably includes proper reporting. The notification of incidents and adverse effects has been essential to implement prevention strategies in medicine or nursing. Without knowing what is really happening and the associated factors, it is not possible to apply effective measures. The SdP culture, which is not based on searching for the guilty professional but on the human factor and the organization of the system, has encouraged the communication of incidents and adverse effects, therefore their analysis and prevention. In physical therapy, the same process of encouraging communication should be applied. AEs associated with physiotherapy is sometimes reported by other health care professionals, such as emergency department doctors. The problem in such cases

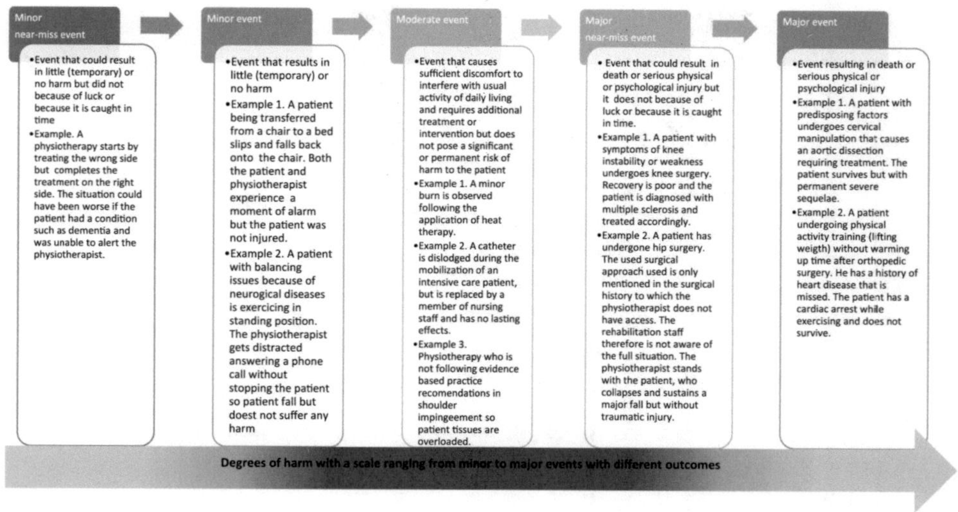

Figure 3.
Continuum of error occurrence with examples from the physiotherapy field. Adapted from Ginsburg et al. [64].

is that reports will probably be incomplete as the attending doctor may not be aware of the patient's history (i.e., the link with physiotherapy) and will not conduct a full root-cause analysis [50].

There is a direct link between the trivialization of possible adverse treatment outcomes and underreporting of errors. Viewing a physiotherapy intervention with inherent risks (however slight) as safe jeopardizes professional autonomy and self-affirmation and impedes acknowledgment of the importance of physiotherapy among other health care professionals and the creation of a culture of safety. It is a vicious circle that needs to be broken if the concept of patient safety is to be integrated into routine physiotherapy practice. Physiotherapy associations and experts in patient safety from other disciplines must strive to foster a culture of patient safety in physiotherapy and lay the bases for the creation of effective systems for reporting incidents, AEs, and near misses. Concerted efforts in this regard should also help reduce the wide variability observed to date [65]. Due to the paucity of evidence on patient safety and physiotherapy and the not well spread consciousness of the situation among the professionals, it is difficult to state which populations receiving physiotherapy are more at risk for medical errors and adverse events in this field.

6. Key directions for the future of patient safety in physiotherapy

Education and training are keys to fostering a culture of safety in physiotherapy [9, 44]. Proper training will ensure correct assessment and inform decisions on when a given treatment is warranted or not. Unfamiliarity with a technique or its potential outcomes could result in injury and should constitute a reason for withholding treatment. Patient safety needs to be incorporated into standard physiotherapy education and training programs, as university graduates receive little or no training in this area. As stated by Boohoo et al. [66] "Many professionals that are performing teaching functions in the health area carry with themselves rich practice baggage from the work environment, with technical knowledge coming from Master and Ph.D. courses,

What you should do in the event of an incident/AE resulting from your or a colleague's conduct • Eliminate as far as possible all immediate dangers to make the situation safe for patients and personnel. • Close off any areas that pose risk. • Alert the necessary authorities (e.g., emergency services). • Arrange for immediate medical assistance. • Report all incidents/AE immediately to minimize the risk of recurrence (inform your manager or another senior person as soon as possible). • Record what happened in the clinical registered history and log the event in the accident/ incident book with a senior member of staff. • Learn from the incident – what was its roo- cause? Could it be prevented from recurring with a different/improved approach? Managers should conduct a new risk assessment and make any necessary amendments to risk management measures to minimize the likelihood of recurrence.	What you should not do in the event of an incident/AE resulting from your or a colleague's conduct • Ignore any concerns you may have. • Engage in or condone poor or illegal practice. • Continue with the same risk. Assessment of existing control measures in place failed. • Fail to put patient health first. • Fail to report or record the event. • Assume someone else will take responsibility. • Fail to follow the procedure in place if it is possible and safe to do so. • Cover up the event or destroy records or evidence. • Engage in an activity that is not permitted by current regulations.
What you should do in the event of an error made by you or a colleague • Report it to your group leader and file a written record. • Assess with your manager whether preventive measures in place were clear enough to have prevented the error re-assess or re-word as necessary. • Learn from the error.	What you should not do in the event of an error made by you or a colleague • Ignore it. • Fail to assess current risk. Assessment/ management plan. • Continue to work in the same way without analyzing what caused the error. • Cover up the error or hide or destroy evidence.

Table 3.
Actions following observation of incidents or adverse effects (AE)s in physiotherapy.

and participation in congresses and scientific events. But this does not mean that they are trained for a systematic approach to error sources and events that may happen in the health care system or that they are concerned with the reporting of events to promote quality improvement processes in the environment where they perform their activities…."

Clinical simulation training is a widely accepted teaching methodology in the health sciences and is recognized by the WHO as a basic and necessary tool. The simulation of real-life clinical scenarios allows participants to practice aspects of their profession, engage in joint discussions and reflections, and transfer lessons learned to the real world. It is based on experiential learning and has been linked to favorable PS outcomes and effective team communication [5, 67].

Systems and strategies for reporting incidents and near-miss events, which account for most errors detected in physiotherapy, are also crucial if progress is to continue. The future of PS in physiotherapy also depends on our ability to transfer awareness and knowledge beyond the hospital setting. Appropriate and inappropriate actions in the event of an incident or near-miss event are summarized in **Table 3**.

7. Conclusions

Thoughtful discussions on the importance of systematic approaches to patient safety are needed in the physiotherapy profession. One key concern should be to gather robust information on the risks associated with physiotherapy practices and explore first-hand experiences through for example, professional societies. Early training in patient safety, particularly in university courses, is also crucial.

Hospital patient safety and quality improvement programs and actions must include physiotherapy and foster awareness of the importance of safety among both physiotherapists and other health care professionals.

It is also necessary to instill a strong patient safety culture outside hospital settings, which is where most physiotherapists practice. Training actions should strive to better visualize near-miss events and facilitate their recognition and systematic reporting to produce data that can be used to develop reliable indicators, foster the growth of patient safety in physiotherapy and heighten awareness of this profession among practitioners from other fields.

The continued idea that standard physiotherapy interventions cause little or no harm is a serious impediment to the detection, reporting, and recording of inherent risks. The key lies in the collection of robust data as only this can drive true change. Finally, professional societies need to foster a culture of patient safety among their members and lay the bases for effective reporting systems and widespread dissemination of near-miss and AE.

Conflict of interest

The authors declare that they have no conflicts of interest. Authors have no financial support to be declared and ethical declarations are not applicable.

Author details

Griselda Gonzalez-Caminal*, Aida Camps Gomez and Carmen Gomar-Sancho
University of Vic-University of Central Catalonia, Manresa, Spain

*Address all correspondence to: ggonzalez@umanresa.cat

References

[1] World Health Organization. What is patient safety?". World Health Organization. 2021. Available at: https://www.who.int/teams/integrated-health-services/patient-safety/about [Accessed May 25, 2022]

[2] Girdler SJ, Girdler JE, Tarpada SP, et al. Nonmaleficence in medical training: Balancing patient care and efficient education. Indian Journal of Medical Ethics. 2019;**4**(2):129-133

[3] Walton M, Kerridge I. Do no harm: Is it time to rethink the Hippocratic Oath? Medical Education. 2014;**48**(1):17-27

[4] Veras M, Kairy D, Paquet N. What is evidence-based physiotherapy? Physiotherapy Canada. 2016;**68**(2):95

[5] Executive Board, 144. Patient safety: Global action on patient safety: Report by the Director-General. 2018. World Health Organization. Available at: https://apps.who.int/iris/handle/10665/327526 [Accessed May 25, 2022]

[6] Rocco C, Garrido A. Seguridad del paciente y cultura de seguridad. Rev. Médica Clínica Las Condes. 2017;**28**(5):785-795

[7] Beecher HK, Todd DP. A study of the deaths associated with anesthesia and surgery: Based on a study of 599, 548 anesthesias in ten institutions 1948-1952, inclusive. Annals of Surgery. 1954;**140**(1):2-35

[8] Kohn L, Corrigan J, Donaldson M. To Err is Human: Building a Safer Health System. 2000. Available at: www.pubmed.ncbi.nlm.nih.gov/25077248 [Accessed May 25, 2022]

[9] WHO. Global patient safety action plan 2021-2030: Towards eliminating avoidable harm in health care. Geneva: World Health Organization. 2021. Available at: https://www.who.int/teams/integrated-health-services/patient-safety/policy/global-patient-safety-action-plan [Accessed May 28, 2022]

[10] Berner ES, Graber ML. Overconfidence as a cause of diagnostic error in medicine. The American Journal of Medicine. 2008;**121**(5 Suppl):S2-S23

[11] Slawomirski L, Auraaen A, Klazinga N. The Economics of Patient Safety: Strengthening a Value-Based Approach to Reducing Patient Harm at National Level. Paris: OECD; 2017. Available from: http://www.oecd.org/els/health-systems/The-economics-of-patient-safety-March-2017.pdf [Accessed May 26, 2022]

[12] Aranaz JM, Aibar C, Vitaller J, Ruiz P. Estudio Nacional sobre los Efectos Adversos ligados a la Hospitalización. ENEAS 2005. Madrid. Ministerio de Sanidad y Consumo. 2006. Available at: https://seguridaddelpaciente.es/resources/contenidos/castellano/2006/ENEAS.pdf [Accessed May 25, 2022]

[13] Ministerio de Sanidad y Política Social/OMS. Estudio IBEAS prevalencia de efectos adversos en hospitales de Latinoamérica. Informes, estudios e investigación 2010. Madrid: Ministerio de Sanidad y Política Social. 2010. Available at: http://bit.ly/2vgnA2y [Accessed May 25, 2022]

[14] Struessel T, Rodriguez JW, Van Zytveld CR. Advocating for a systems approach to enhance patient safety in physical therapy practice: A clinical commentary. HPA Resource. 2017;**17**:1

[15] Alcântara FA. Perception of physiotherapists on bioethical aspects

in palliative care. Revista Bioética. 2021;**29**:107-114

[16] Sturm A, Edwards I, Fryer CE, et al. (Almost) 50 shades of an ethical situation — international physiotherapists' experiences of everyday ethics: A qualitative analysis. Physiotherapy Theory and Practice. 2022;**4**:1-18

[17] King J, Anderson CM. Patient safety and physiotherapy: What does it mean for your clinical practice? Physiotherapy Canada. 2010;**62**(3):172-175

[18] Paul A, Mullerpatan R. Review of physiotherapy awareness across the globe. International Journal of Health Science and Research. 2015;**5**(10):294-301

[19] Ebenezer C, Goh CXH, Jemeela S, et al. Awareness and knowledge of physiotherapy among medical and health sciences students: A Cross-Sectional Study. Research Journal of Pharmaceutical and Technology. 2019;**12**(4):1695-1706

[20] Goodwin R, Moffatt F, Hendrick P, et al. First point of contact physiotherapy; a qualitative study. Physiotherapy. 2020;**108**:29-36

[21] World Confederation of Physical Therapy. Description of physical therapy Policy statement. 2019. Available at: https://world.physio/policy/ps-descriptionPT [Accessed June 02, 2022]

[22] Higgs J, Refshauge K, Ellis E. Portrait of the physiotherapy profession. Journal of Interprofessional Care. 2000;**15**(1):79-89

[23] Mak S, Hunt M, Boruff J, et al. Exploring professional identity in rehabilitation professions: A scoping review. Advances in Health Sciences Education. 2022;**27**(3):793-815

[24] Hon S, Ritter R, Allen DD. Cost-effectiveness and outcomes of direct access to physical therapy for musculoskeletal disorders compared to physician-first access in the United States: Systematic review and meta-analysis. Physical Therapy. 2021;**101**(1):pzaa201

[25] Demont A, Bourmaud A, Kechichian A, et al. The impact of direct access physiotherapy compared to primary care physician led usual care for patients with musculoskeletal disorders: A systematic review of the literature. Disability and Rehabilitation. 2021;**43**(12):1637-1648

[26] McCallum CA, DiAngelis T. Direct access: Factors that affect physical therapist practice in the state of Ohio. Physical Therapy. 2012;**92**(5):688-706

[27] Gibson BE. A post-critical physiotherapy ethics: A commitment to openness. In: Gibson BE, Nicholls D, Setchell J, et al., editors. Manipulating Practices: A Critical Physiotherapy Reader. Oslo: Cappelen Damm; 2018. pp. 35-54. DOI: 10.23865/noasp.29

[28] World Confederation of Physical Therapy. Ethical principles and the responsibilities of physiotherapists and member organizations Description of physical therapy Policy statement. 2022. Available at: https://world.physio/sites/default/files/2022-03/PS-2022-Ethical_responsibilities_principles_Eng.pdf [Accessed June 02, 2022]

[29] Struessel T, Forster JE, Van Zytveld C. Doctor of physical therapy student experiences during clinical education: Patient safety, error, and the system. Journal, Physical Therapy Education. 2019;**33**(1):3-15

[30] Bordas-Martínez J, Luzardo-González A, Arencibia A, et al. Effects

of early physical therapy and follow-up in acute severe coronavirus disease 2019 pneumonia: A Retrospective Observational Study. Frontiers in Medicine. 2022;**9**:866055

[31] Goñi-Viguria R, Yoldi-Arzoz E, Casajús-Sola L, et al. Respiratory physiotherapy in intensive care unit: Bibliographic review. Enfermería Intensiva (English ed.). 2018;**29**(4):168-181

[32] Newman AN, Gravesande J, Rotella S, et al. Physiotherapy in the neurotrauma intensive care unit: A scoping review. Journal of Critical Care. 2018;**48**:390-406

[33] Perreault K, Dionne CE, Rossignol M, et al. Physiotherapy practice in the private sector: Organizational characteristics and models. BMC Health Services Research. 2014;**14**(1):1-13

[34] Sandstrom R. Malpractice by physical therapists: Danalysis of reports in the National Practitioner Data Bank public use data file 1991-2004. Journal of Allied Health. 2007;**36**(4):201-208

[35] Studdert DM, Mello MM, Brennan TA. Medical malpractice. The New England Journal of Medicine. 2004;**350**:3

[36] Di Luca A, Vetrugno G, Pascali VL, et al. Perspectives on patient safety and medical malpractice. Journal of Patient Safety. 2019;**15**(4):e78-e81

[37] Reisch LM, Flores MJ, Radick AC, et al. Malpractice and patient safety concerns. American Journal of Clinical Pathology. 2020;**154**(5):700-707

[38] Pawlson LG, O'Kane ME. Malpractice prevention, patient safety, and quality of care: A critical linkage. The American Journal of Managed Care. 2004;**10**(4):281-284

[39] Reason J. Human Error. Boston: Cambridge University Press; 1990

[40] Emanuel L, Berwick D, Conway J, et al. What exactly is patient safety? Journal of Medical Regulation. 2009;**95**(1):13-24

[41] Saks MJ, Landsman S. Does malpractice liability make healthcare safer? Aligning law and policy with evidence. Wake Forest Journal of Law Policy. 2022;**12**:205-257

[42] Van Zytveld CR, Rodriguez JW, Struessel TS. Lessons learned from a major near miss: A case report including recommendations to improve future patient safety in rehabilitation. Internet Journal of Allied Health Science and Practice. 2016;**14**(3):Article 5

[43] Kachalia A, Mello MM, Nallamothu BK, et al. Legal and policy interventions to improve patient safety. Circulation. 2016;**133**(7):661-671

[44] Scheirton LS, Mu K, Lohman H, et al. Error and patient safety: Ethical analysis of cases in occupational and physical therapy practice. Medicine, Health Care, and Philosophy. 2007;**10**(3):301

[45] Boyce D, Wempe H, Campbell C, et al. Adverse events associated with the therapeutic dry needling. International Journal of Sports Physical Therapy. 2020;**15**(1):103-113

[46] Carlesso LC, Cairney J, Dolovich L, et al. Defining adverse events in manual therapy: An exploratory qualitative analysis of the patient perspective. Manual Therapy. 2011;**16**(5):440-446

[47] Krein SL, Abdul-Wahab Y, Kadri R, et al. Adverse events experienced by participants in a back pain walking intervention: A descriptive study. Chronic Illness. 2016;**12**(1):71-80

[48] Carlesso LC, Macdermid JC, Santaguida PL, et al. Determining adverse events in patients with neck pain receiving orthopedic manual physiotherapy: A pilot and feasibility study. Physiotherapy Canada. 2013;**65**(3):255-265

[49] Carlesso LC, Gross AR, Santaguida PL, et al. Adverse events associated with the use of cervical manipulation and mobilization for the treatment of neck pain in adults: A systematic review. Manual Therapy. 2010;**15**(5):434-444

[50] Puentedura EJ, O'Grady WH. Safety of thrust joint manipulation in the thoracic spine: A systematic review. The Journal of Manual & Manipulative Therapy. 2015;**23**(3):154-161

[51] Swait G, Finch R. What are the risks of manual treatment of the spine? A scoping review for clinicians. Chiropractic and Manual Therapy. 2017:25-37. DOI: 10.1186/s12998-017-0168-5

[52] Ghosh M, O'Connell B, Afrifa-Yamoah E, et al. A retrospective cohort study of factors associated with severity of falls in hospital patients. Scientific Reports. 2022;**12**:12,266

[53] Nydahl P, Sricharoenchai T, Chandra S, et al. Safety of patient mobilization and rehabilitation in the intensive care unit. Systematic review with meta-analysis. Annals of the American Thoracic Society. 2017;**14**(5):766-777

[54] Mayer KP, Joseph-Isang E, Robinson LE, et al. Safety and feasibility of physical rehabilitation and active mobilization in patients requiring continuous renal replacement therapy: A systematic review. Critical Care Medicine. 2020;**48**(11):e1112

[55] Maltser S, Cristian A, Silver JK, a. A focused review of safety considerations in cancer rehabilitation. PM & R : The Journal of Injury, Function, and Rehabilitation. 2017;**9**(9 Suppl 2):S415-S428

[56] Vetrovsky T, Steffl M, Stastny P, et al. The efficacy and safety of lower-limb plyometric training in older adults: A systematic review. Sports Medical Aucklan and Newzealand. 2019;**49**(1):113-131

[57] Raney NH, Petersen EJ, Smith TA, et al. Development of a clinical prediction rule to identify patients with neck pain likely to benefit from cervical traction and exercise. European Spine Journal. 2009;**18**:382-391

[58] Butler DS. Neuro Orthopedic Group. The Neurodynamic Techniques: A Definitive Guide from the Noigroup Team. 1st ed. Adelaida: Noigroup Publications; 2005. p. 98

[59] Maitland GD. Maitland's Vertebral Manipulation. Oxford: Butterworth-Heinemann; 2001. p. p480

[60] Brennan MT, Green M, Gomes B, et al. Professional liability insurance in Canada: How insurance by physiotherapists, for physiotherapists' supports excellence in practice. Physiotherapy. 2015;**101**:e170-e171

[61] Kilner E, Sheppard LA. The role of teamwork and communication in the emergency department: A systematic review. International Emergency Nursing. 2010;**18**(3):127-137

[62] Hegarty J, Flaherty SJ, Saab MM, et al. An international perspective on definitions and terminology used to describe serious reportable patient safety incidents: A systematic review. Journal of Patient Safety. 2021;**17**(8):e1247-e1254

[63] Yang Y, Liu H. The effect of patient safety culture on nurses' near-miss reporting intention: The moderating role of perceived severity of near misses. Journal of Research in Nursing. 2021;**26**(1-2):6-16

[64] Ginsburg LR, Chuang YT, Richardson J, et al. Categorizing errors and adverse events for learning: A provider perspective. Healthcare. 2009;**12**:154-160

[65] Puentedura E, March J, Anders J, et al. Safety of cervical spine manipulation: Are adverse events preventable and are manipulations being performed appropriately? A review of 134 case reports. The Journal of Manual & Manipulative Therapy. 2012;**20**(2):66-74

[66] Bohomol E, de Freitas MA. Ensino da segurança do paciente na graduação em saúde: reflexões sobre saberes e fazeres. Interface - Comun Saúde Educ. 2016;**20**(58):727-741

[67] Freytag J, Stroben F, Hautz WE, et al. Improving patient safety through better teamwork: How effective are different methods of simulation debriefing? Protocol for a pragmatic, prospective and randomized study. BMJ Open. 2017;7(6):e015977

Chapter 9

Patient Safety and Healthcare Worker Safety in Gastrointestinal Endoscopy during COVID-19 Pandemic

Rabbinu Rangga Pribadi

Abstract

Patient safety remains a concern worldwide. Failure in executing patient safety measures will result in serious consequences such as diminished patient's quality of life, increased morbidity and mortality, increased negative image, and public distrust of healthcare providers. Healthcare worker (HW) safety is also increasingly becoming a concern. During the COVID-19 pandemic, we should implement standards including COVID-19 screening, patient safety, healthcare worker safety, endoscopy room, equipment, and personal protective equipment (PPE). This review is intended to discuss the preparation before, during, and after gastrointestinal endoscopy (GIE) procedures to ensure patient and healthcare worker safety in the era of the COVID-19 pandemic. A literature search was conducted from August 2022 to October 2022 and comprised several journals related to the topic. The literatures were searched on credible platforms such as Google Scholar, PubMed, and Science Direct. Most of the endoscopy units were reducing the performance, down to 50%–90% reductions. The units prioritized cases using time-sensitive factors to urgent, semi-urgent, and elective classification. The endoscopy procedure is performed in accordance with protocols to maintain patient and healthcare worker safety. Adherence of gastrointestinal endoscopy procedure strictly to standards has to be implemented to protect patient and healthcare workers during COVID-19 pandemic.

Keywords: gastrointestinal endoscopy, patient safety, healthcare worker safety

1. Introduction

Patient safety is an important global issue. It serves as the basis of safe and optimal medical care worldwide [1, 2]. World Health Organization (WHO) defines patient safety as "A framework of organized activities that creates cultures, processes, procedures, behaviors, technologies and environments in health care that consistently and sustainably lower risks, reduce the occurrence of avoidable harm, make errors less likely and reduce the impact of harm when it does occur" [2, 3].

Patient safety forms the foundation of the best practice in providing high-quality medical service. Failure to implement patient safety measures will generate serious consequences such as decreased patient's quality of life, increased morbidity and mortality, increased negative image, and public distrust of healthcare providers. Those situations that may cause or already caused unnecessary harm to the patient are described as incidents [4]. According to WHO, patient safety incidents are classified into three groups: near miss, harmful incidents, and no-harm incidents. Harmful incidents are further divided into two types: adverse events and adverse reactions [3].

The importance of healthcare worker (HW) safety has been increasingly recognized as well, especially after the declaration of the COVID-19 pandemic. Healthcare worker safety is closely interconnected to patient safety [5]. Improving the use of personal protective equipment (PPE) and reporting-analyzing serious safety-related incidents are the most relevant aspects of gastrointestinal endoscopy (GIE) [6].

Gastrointestinal endoscopy (GIE) is one of the fastest-growing procedures, and patient safety undeniably forms the foundation of delivering high-quality GIE. However, patient safety issues are still reported. Correa, et al. [4] stated that there were 111 incidents out of 42,863 (0.25%) GIE procedures in Brazil's tertiary hospitals. The percentage of near misses, no-harm incidents, and adverse event cases were 34.2%, 40.5%, and 23.4%, respectively. Incorrect patient identification was the most prevalent incident [4].

In the early days of the COVID-19 pandemic, GIE practices declined as endoscopists were concerned about SARS-CoV-2 infection. Zein et al. [7] reported that 56.5% of Indonesian GI endoscopists temporarily stopped their endoscopy practice. Han et al. [8] showed that in South Korea, endoscopists decided to perform a limited number of GIE. Endoscopic procedures should be performed with safety precautions for patients and also healthcare workers [9]. Rashid emphasized that the endoscopy unit should be reorganized to facilitate procedures as safely as possible along with general measures and COVID-19 screening [10].

2. Methodology

A narrative review approach was used for evidence synthesis. The current format allowed a comprehensive approach to gain a thorough understanding of the patient and healthcare workers' safety issues. A literature search was conducted during August 2022 and October 2022 and comprised several journals related to the topic. The literatures were searched on credible platforms such as Google Scholar, PubMed, and Science Direct. After further reading and screening, articles related to the topic were narrowed to the specific area of discussion.

3. Safety in GI endoscopy

Gastrointestinal endoscopy procedures should be adjusted to ensure both patient and healthcare worker safety. Many countries have developed their endoscopy management to improve the national quality of endoscopy procedures. In South Korea, The Korean Society of Gastrointestinal Endoscopy (KSGE) has initiated the National Endoscopy Quality Improvement Program to manage programs on endoscopic procedures, includes qualification of endoscopists, improvement of instruments and facilities in endoscopy units, and measurement of outcomes of endoscopy screening [11].

According to World Health Organization (WHO), recommendations to prevent harm during endoscopy include prevention of harm from anesthesia, avoidance of allergic or adverse drug reactions, effective communication among healthcare providers, standardized reporting on procedures, results, and complications [12].

In the era of the COVID-19 pandemic, both patients undergoing GIE and healthcare workers performing GIE are at risk of acquiring infection via direct contact, aerosol, or contaminated body fluid [8]. Most of the endoscopy units were reducing the performance, down to 50–90% reductions. The units prioritized the case using urgent, semi-urgent, and elective classifications [13]. Gastrointestinal endoscopy is performed only on potentially life-threatening conditions (urgent), such as gastrointestinal bleeding, foreign body retrieval, urgent nutritional access, cancer patient, and other conditions that cannot be postponed [9, 10].

To minimize the risk of COVID-19 transmission, some strategies and modifications need to be implemented. To begin with, pre-endoscopic modifications are patient evaluation, COVID-19 screening, healthcare worker (HW) well-being, endoscopy room, equipment, and PPE. While the endoscopic modifications are PPE and restriction in the number of involved healthcare workers in the procedure room during endoscopy. Finally, the post-endoscopic adjustment is recovery room, endoscopic room decontamination, and scope disinfection.

4. Patient safety

Patient safety incidents may occur mostly because of individual error, suboptimal team performance, or task-related problems. Even though the incidents are usually to have minor or do not need immediate treatment, it also has to be prevented for the patients' safety [14].

Patient misidentification is of utmost concern. In 2003, the Joint Commission International (JCI) emphasized patient identification as the first International Patient Safety Goals (IPSG). Adverse events due to treatment errors, transfusion errors, testing errors, and wrong-person procedures mostly stemmed from patient misidentification [15].

Patient safety incidents are varying widely, which may occur on arrival, procedure, or even recovery from sedation. Studies have shown that half of the significant adverse events in GIE are associated with sedation [16]. In 2021, Correa et al. [4] revealed that 40.1%, 24.6%, and 35.3% of all incidents consisted of events that occurred before, during, and after procedures, respectively. The study evaluated 50% of adverse events that occur during and after procedures were due to gastrointestinal perforation and gastrointestinal laceration/bleeding without perforation, 19.2% due to skin lesions, and 11.5% due to falls [4].

Checklist by WHO showed the ability to reduce mortality from 1.5% to 0.8%. It will not prevent every error in GIE, but it can minimize incidents and encourage a culture of safety through improved teamwork in the endoscopy room. It is a simple, inexpensive, and effective tool that has the potential to promote safe GIE procedures [14].

5. COVID-19 screening

Before patients enter the endoscopy room, they should be evaluated. COVID-19 screening and body temperature checking are mandatory. The screening will determine the next step. Symptoms such as fever, respiratory problems, and cough will lead healthcare workers to postpone the procedure and transfer the patient to an infectious disease clinic or emergency department for further treatment.

All patients who will undergo GIE should be tested with a SARS-CoV-2 reverse transcriptase polymerase chain reaction (RT-PCR) swab [10]. According to American Gastroenterological Association (AGA), the suggested testing is nucleic acid examination such as NAAT or rapid RT-PCR for an endoscopy center that implements pre-endoscopic SARS-CoV-2 testing [17]. One study showed that SARS-CoV-2 RT-PCR examination is an effective approach to resume GIE practice in the United States. They recommended that PCR testing should be employed during the pandemic's second phase [18]. Some experts also recommend the chest CT scan because the result may come out first than the RT-PCR SARS-CoV-2 test, but later findings showed that non-severe COVID-19 patients have no radiographic abnormality displayed, so chest CT has limited value in screening for COVID-19 prior to endoscopy [9, 10].

Healthcare workers in the endoscopy unit must take the right and thoughtful decision regarding the urgency of the patient's condition. Urgent patients are related to time-sensitive factors that if the procedure is postponed, then a higher risk of threat to the patient is inevitable (**Figure 1**). To make it easier, experts recommend using these questions to answer: is the procedure indicated, is the procedure time sensitive, if yes, it has to be done within 2 weeks or 8 weeks, if not time-sensitive, the procedure can be delayed after 8 weeks (**Figure 2**). In a different study, the classification of the patient condition is divided into three conditions: emergent condition must be performed within 1 week; the urgent condition is performed within 1–8 weeks, and non-time-sensitive can be delayed for more than 8 weeks [19]. This action has to consider the patient's medical records, laboratory results, cross-sectional images, and endoscopic reports [9, 20].

The urgent indication has been classified by some studies and includes gastrointestinal bleeding, perforation treatment, stent insertion for gastrointestinal obstruction, biliary sepsis, acute cholangitis, and other conditions, which met the criteria of an urgent situation. Semi-urgent patient includes endoscopic therapy for neoplasia such

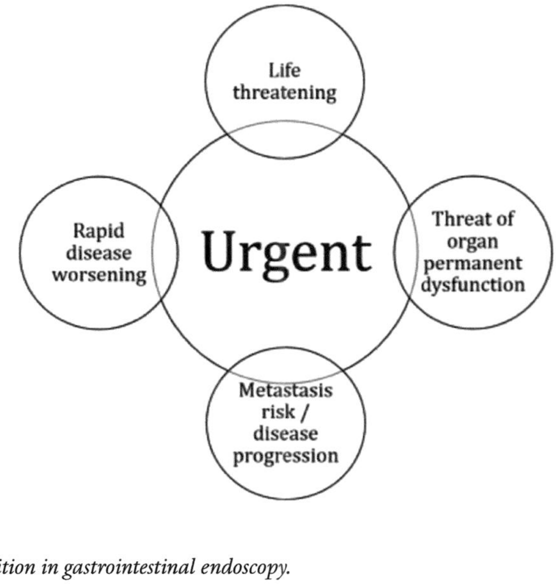

Figure 1.
Criteria of urgent condition in gastrointestinal endoscopy.

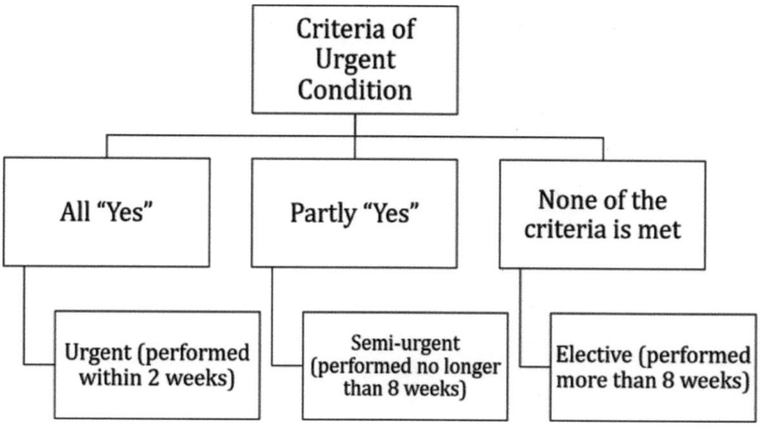

Figure 2.
Prioritization of gastrointestinal endoscopy.

as polypectomy, endoscopic mucosal resection or dissection, occult gastrointestinal bleeding, enteroscopy, and endoscopic retrograde cholangiopancreatography (ERCP) for pancreatobiliary malignancy. If the COVID-19 patient's condition is not urgent, then the GIE procedure will be delayed for at least 14 days or after negative RT-PCR testing [9, 20].

The patients who will undergo endoscopy procedure need to fill out the form of travel history, close contact with suspected or confirmed COVID-19 persons, and informed consent for GIE procedure [9]. The consent must be clear and include all procedures and interventions that will be taken or reduced during endoscopy [20]. The patients have to wear a surgical mask and perform hand hygiene; some also recommend wearing gloves. While waiting, the patients are encouraged to minimize close contact and communication. Patients can be accompanied by one adult and no visitors are allowed (**Figure 3**) [10].

6. Patient evaluation

The preparation and precautions for endoscopy procedure are essential for patient safety. In order to reduce incidents, every patient should be comprehensively evaluated before GIE. The American Society of Gastrointestinal Endoscopy (ASGE) recommended that the initial endoscopic procedure is confirming the correct patient and procedure to be performed [21].

Before performing an endoscopic procedure, the patient's identity should be checked. Name and date of birth should be asked and checked on patients' wristband and medical record or document. The recommendations are confirming the patient by checking a minimum of two data: name and date of birth. The indication and type of the planned procedure should also be verified. The medical personnel, who will perform GIE, needs to deliver essential and relevant information related to the procedure to the patient. Informed consent has to be delivered in every endoscopy procedure [22].

Medical history might affect tolerance to the procedure. Patients' medical history needs to be checked thoroughly for the patient undergoing without sedation or with sedation, especially in moderate/deep sedation. The medical history will show the

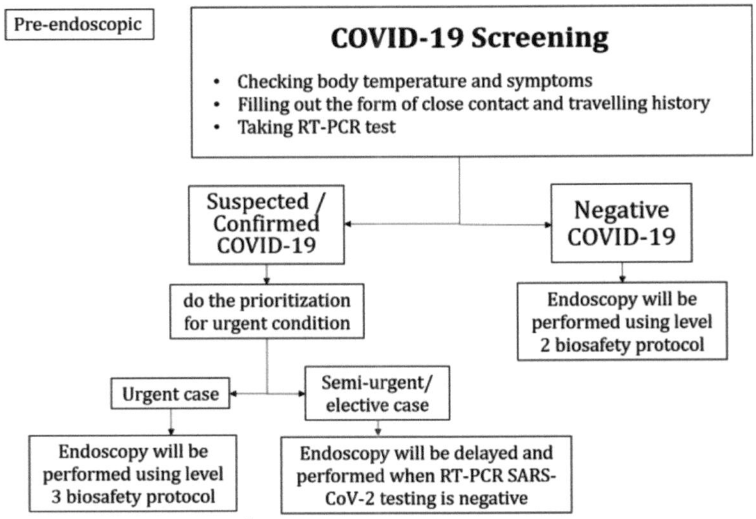

Figure 3.
Workflow of gastrointestinal endoscopy using COVID-19 screening.

presence of respiratory, cardiovascular, neurologic, renal, or other problems [22]. History of obstructive sleep apnea may predict ventilatory function disturbance with sedation [23]. Physical examination should be done, including vital signs, auscultation of the heart and lungs, a baseline level of consciousness, and assessment of airways [22].

7. Healthcare worker safety

Healthcare worker well-being is one pillar that contributes to patient safety [5]. It comprised physical and mental aspects. Healthcare workers should be protected from medical hazards. Standard PPE should be provided by the hospital. Vaccination programs including COVID-19 immunization should be given to all HW. Personal hygiene such as regular handwashing should be enforced according to the WHO protocol [5, 10]. Healthcare workers are working in high-demand and high-risk medical environments in which psychological stress can occur. Their mental problems should be addressed. Psychological support should be provided to ensure HW's well-being [10].

COVID-19 patients are admitted to hospitals with various comorbidities, including GI diseases. Those patients might require GIE for the evaluation and management of digestive diseases [17]. Gastrointestinal endoscopy procedures pose a transmission risk to the HW (endoscopist and endoscopic nurses). Body fluids from COVID-19 patients can spread during the procedure. Saliva can contaminate the pillow during esophagogastroduodenoscopy (EGD), and feces may contaminate the bed during colonoscopy. Prevention of infection to HW is important [24, 25].

The Indonesian Society for Digestive Endoscopy (ISDE) has released a particular recommendation for performing GIE during the COVID-19 pandemic. Their recommendations consisted of patient selection, selection of endoscopy room, medical staff protection, recovery room, and equipment disinfection. The highlights of these recommendations are defined as whether the patient has an indication for urgent, semi-urgent, or elective GIE. It is mandatory to limit the indications for GIE only for emergencies such as acute gastrointestinal bleeding, foreign bodies impaction, acute cholangitis, and cancer care only. All elective cases should be postponed to reduce the SARS-CoV-2 transmission [9].

To minimize the cross-infection, the number of involved HW is recommended to be restricted in endoscopy procedures. The HW should remain to stay in the endoscopy room until the procedure is finished and avoids encountering other staff. The staff restrictions also can be an effective way to wear PPE efficiently, since it is the commodity that is in great demand during the COVID-19 pandemic [10, 26].

8. Personal protective equipment

Personal protective equipment (PPE) is equipment specially designed to protect the HW or other employees who wear it to improve their personal safety against infectious materials. There are various PPE components including masks, gloves, gowns, goggles, face shields, disposable hair caps, and shoe covers [27].

GI endoscopy units have to define the policies in which PPE should be worn during certain exposure. In low-risk exposure, which has no direct contact with contaminated devices, body fluid, and other infectious substances, HW should wear minimum components of PPE (mask, gown, and glove). However, in the high-risk procedure, which has direct contact with a contaminated device, body fluid, and needs direct treatment, HW must wear the full component of PPE. Every personnel has to understand how to do PPE donning and doffing appropriately [27, 28]. Personal protective equipment will be effective if supported with other preventive actions, such as physical distancing, hand wash, and disinfection of medical equipment [26].

When performing GIE in suspected or confirmed COVID-19 patients, the involved HW should wear level 3 biosafety PPE. Those are N95 masks, coverall suits, hair caps, face shields, double gloves, and boots. Prolonged use of N95 for up to 4 hours is tolerable. Level 2 biosafety PPE is recommended to wear for endoscopic staff who performed negative or low-risk COVID-19. The equipment for level 2 includes an N95/FFP2/FFP3 mask, disposable waterproof gown, goggles, caps, and shoe covers. All HWs should be educated to wear proper PPE according to standards to minimize infection because the infection potentially occurs during donning and doffing PPE [9, 29].

In a study related to PPE in GIE procedure, most HW implemented proper hygiene, yet they are not educated enough to perform PPE donning and doffing [13]. The HWs have to discard used PPE properly to the waste container and continue with washing hands and other open body parts after the procedure is done [28].

9. Endoscopy room and equipment

The separation of clean and contaminated rooms should be implemented for the endoscopy room, sign-in room, and recovery room. One-way flow for equipment and patients is the recommended approach [10]. The traffic flow in the endoscopy room should be organized to make efficient and easy movement for patient, HW, and any equipment needed. It also prevents any infection or contamination within the room [30].

The size of the endoscopy room is determined by the complexity of the procedure. A procedure such as ERCP, which needed specialized equipment, requires bigger space. The room has to have enough space and supporting facilities for vital equipment such as oxygen source, suction source, and uninterruptible power supply. The room needs to be checked and monitored periodically even in the external aspect such as temperature and humidity [28]. The recovery room also needs to have appropriate spaces and provide comfortable conditions that can keep the patient's privacy [28].

For suspected or confirmed COVID-19, GIE is recommended to be performed in a negative pressure room [29]. Endoscopy room surfaces and floor should be disinfected using chlorine after the procedure. New and clean bed sheets should be provided. The endoscopes should be disinfected according to standard protocol [10].

Ventilation in the endoscopy room is important since SARS-CoV-2 spreads into the air. The virus may spread in aerosol-generating procedures such as EGD or ERCP. Negative pressure rooms can prevent the aerosol-containing virus to spread wider in the air. If negative pressure rooms are not available, then portable high-efficiency particulate air (HEPA) filters may be a reasonable alternative [9].

After the procedure is completed, patients will be directed into a recovery room. The patient is provided with a surgical mask and other PPEs depending on their COVID-19 status. It is also recommended to differentiate among patients to prevent cross-infections of COVID-19. The staff who cleaned used equipment and room has to wear PPE including a head cap, gown, surgical mask, face shield, shoe covers, and gloves, since they will be cleaning and potentially contacting with scopes, surfaces, and equipment after procedures [10, 24].

SARS-CoV-2 is reported to be cleared using disinfectant containing hydrogen peroxide, alcohol, and chlorine. Any high-contacted surface and equipment have to be disinfected after each endoscopic procedure. Ultraviolet irradiation and ozone treatment can be advanced sterilization methods in an endoscopy room [10]. The frequency of disinfection can differ regarding the risk of the patient's status. In suspected or confirmed COVID-19 patients (high-risk), at least two times disinfection processing is suggested to minimize contamination; meanwhile, in negative COVID-19 patients (low-risk), it can be done once according to the applicable standard [9].

10. Conclusion

Adherence of GIE procedures strictly to guidelines should be implemented to protect patients and HW during the COVID-19 pandemic. Healthcare workers' well-being and safety are also a priority that cannot be neglected. The COVID-19 pandemic is still unpredictable, so it will need more innovations and dynamic regulations to overcome the problem.

Author details

Rabbinu Rangga Pribadi
Division of Gastroenterology, Pancreatobiliary and Digestive Endoscopy, Department of Internal Medicine, Faculty of Medicine Universitas Indonesia, Cipto Mangunkusumo National General Hospital, Jakarta, Indonesia

*Address all correspondence to: rabbinurangga@gmail.com

References

[1] World Health Organization. Implications of the COVID-19 Pandemic for Patient Safety: A Rapid Review. Geneva: World Health Organization; 2022. pp. 1-49. License: CC BY-NC-SA 3.0 IGO

[2] World Health Organization. Global Patient Safety Action Plan 2021-2030: Towards Eliminating Avoidable Harm in Health Care. Geneva: World Health Organization; 2021. pp. 1689-1699. License: CC BY-NC-SA 3.0 IGO

[3] World Health Organization. Patient Safety Incident Reporting and Learning Systems: Technical Report and Guidance. Geneva: World Health Organization; 2020. pp. 1-51. License: CC BY-NC-SA 3.0 IGO

[4] Correa CSM, Bagatini A, Prates CG, Sander GB. Patient safety in an endoscopy unit: An observational retrospective analysis of reported incidents. Brazilian Journal of Anesthesiology (English Ed.). 2021;**71**(2):137-141

[5] World Health Organization. Charter: Health Worker Safety: A Priority for Patient Safety. World Health Organization; 2020. pp. 1-6. Available from: https://apps.who.int/iris/handle/10665/339287. License: CC BY-NC-SA 3.0 IGO

[6] Binns C, Low WY. World patient safety day. Asia-Pacific Journal of Public Health. 2020;**32**(6-7):300-301

[7] Zein AFMZ, Pribadi RR, Khasanah U, Bestari MB, Syam AF. Clinical gastroenterology and gastrointestinal endoscopy practices during the coronavirus disease 2019 pandemic in Indonesia: An Online Nationwide Survey. Clinical Endoscopy. 2021;**2021**:1-8

[8] Han J, Kim EY. Sharing our experience of operating an endoscopy unit in the midst of a covid-19 outbreak. Clinical Endoscopy. 2020;**53**(2):243-245

[9] Maulahela H, Syam AF, Renaldi K, Bestari MB, Sutikno R, Abdullah M, et al. A clinical and procedural guideline for gastrointestinal endoscopy units during COVID-19 pandemic era. Acta Medica Indonesiana. 2020;**52**(4):431-435

[10] Lui RN. Safety in endoscopy for patients and healthcare workers during the COVID-19 pandemic. Techniques and Innovations in Gastrointestinal Endoscopy. 2021;**23**:170-178

[11] Jung Y, Kim JW, Im JP, Cho YK, Lee TH, Jang JY. Safety of gastrointestinal endoscopy in Korea: A Nationwide Survey and Population-Based Study. Journal of Korean Medical Science. 2022;**37**(4):1-11

[12] Anderson J, Bensoussan Y, Townsley R, Kell E. In-Office endoscopic laryngeal laser procedures: A patient safety initiative. Otolaryngology. 2018;**159**(1):136-142

[13] Alboraie M, Piscoya A, Tran QT, Mendelsohn RB, Butt AS, Lenz L, et al. The global impact of COVID-19 on gastrointestinal endoscopy units: An international survey of endoscopists. Arabian Journal of Gastroenterology. 2020;**21**(3):156-161

[14] Matharoo M, Thomas-Gibson S, Haycock A, Sevdalis N. Implementation of an endoscopy safety checklist. Frontline in Gastroenterology. 2014;**5**(4):260-265

[15] Abdellatif A, Bagian JP, Barajas ER, Cohen M, Cousins D, Denham CR, et al.

Patient identification: Patient safety solutions, volume 1, solution 2, May 2007. The Joint Commission Journal on Quality and Patient Safety [Internet]. 2007;**33**(7):434-437

[16] Aisenberg J. Endoscopic sedation: Equipment and personnel. Gastrointestinal Endoscopy Clinics of North America. 2008;**18**:641-649

[17] Sultan S, Siddique S, Singh S, Altayar O, Caliendo AM, Davitkov P, et al. AGA rapid review and guideline for SARS-CoV2 testing and endoscopy post-vaccination: 2021Update. Gastroenterologia;**2021**:1011-1029

[18] Corral JE, Hoogenboom SA, Kröner PT, Vazquez-roque MI. COVID-19 polymerase chain reaction testing before endoscopy: An economic analysis. Gastrointestinal Endoscopy. 2020;**92**(January):524-534

[19] Feuerstein JD, Bilal M, Berzin TM, Calderwood AH, Guturu P, Juncadella AC, et al. Since January 2020 Elsevier has created a COVID-19 resource centre with free information in English and Mandarin on the novel coronavirus COVID- 19. The COVID-19 resource centre is hosted on Elsevier Connect, the company' s public news and information website. Elsevier hereby grants permission to make all its COVID-19-related research that is available on the COVID-19 resource centre - including this research content - immediately available in PubMed Central and other publicly funded repositories , such as the WHO COVID database with rights for unrestricted research re-use and analyses in any form or by any means with acknowledgement of the original source. These permissions are Triage of General Gastrointestinal Endoscopic Procedures During the COVID-19 Pandemic: Results From a National Delphi Consensus Panel. 2020;(January)

[20] MacHicado JD, Papachristou GI, Cote GA, Wani S, Groce JR, Conwell DL, et al. Pancreaticobiliary endoscopy in the COVID-19 pandemic era. Pancreas. 2020;**49**(6):729-732

[21] Raphael K, Cerrone S, Sceppa E, Schneider P, Laumenede T, Lynch A, et al. Improving patient safety in the endoscopy unit: Utilization of remote video auditing to improve time-out compliance. Gastrointestinal Endoscopy. 2019;**90**(3):424-429

[22] Kang SH, Hyun JJ. Preparation and patient evaluation for safe Gastrointestinal Endoscopy. Clinical Endoscopy. 2013;**46**(3):212-218

[23] Mitty RD, Wild DM. The pre- and postprocedure assessment of patients undergoing sedation for gastrointestinal endoscopy. Gastrointestinal Endoscopy Clinics of North America. 2008;**18**(4):627-640

[24] Leddin D, Armstrong D, Ali RAR, Barkun A, Butt AS, Chen Y, et al. Personal protective equipment for endoscopy in low-resource settings during the COVID-19 pandemic guidance from the World Gastroenterology Organisation. Journal of Clinical Gastroenterology. 2020;**54**(10):833-840

[25] Galloro G, Pisani A, Maurizio R, Lamazza A, Cengia G, Ciliberto E, et al. Elsevier has created a COVID-19 resource centre with free information in English and Mandarin on the novel coronavirus COVID- 19. The COVID-19 resource centre is hosted on Elsevier Connect, the company' s public news and information. Digestive and Liver Disease. 2020, 2020;**52**(January):800-807

[26] Dhir V. Personal protective equipment use for gastrointestinal endoscopy: Are we ready? Journal of Digestive Endoscopy. 2020;**11**(01):53-54

[27] Mathew S, Philip M. Personal protective equipment during endoscopy. Journal of Digestive Endoscopy. 2020;**11**:45-52

[28] Calderwood AH, Chapman FJ, Cohen J, Cohen LB, Collins J, Day LW, et al. Guidelines for safety in the gastrointestinal endoscopy unit. Gastrointestinal Endoscopy. 2014;**79**(3):363-372

[29] Pribadi RR, Pitarini UA, Muzellina VN, Aziza NS, Maulahela H, Renaldi K, et al. Clinical practice of gastrointestinal endoscopy in COVID-19 patients: An experience from Indonesia. Clinical Endoscopy. 2022;**55**:156-159

[30] Deas T, Sinsel L. Ensuring patient safety and optimizing efficiency during gastrointestinal endoscopy. AORN Journal. 2014;**99**(3):396-406

Chapter 10

Prevention Strategies for Patient Safety in Hospitals: Methodical Paradigm, Managerial Perspective, and Artificial Intelligence Advancements

Sunil Jain, Bhagya Kamal Jain, Prem Kamal Jain and Arvind Singh Kushwaha

Abstract

Patient safety is fundamental to high-quality patient care. Hospitalization has its inherent complications. Medical errors can further comprise patient safety. Hospitals provides an opportunity for practicing preventive medicine. Two important areas are (i) making treatment and hospitalization free from side-effects (ii) obviating medical errors. In hospitals these can have serious consequences. Patient safety compromise can occur at the individual or system level. A methodical model for this should include (i) Intervention design (ii) Intervention implementation (iii) Intervention institutionalization. Managerial perspective important for leadership and team work. Leadership can energize excellence in the coordination and mobilization of the large number of inter-dependent processes and resources needed for achievement of patient safety. Three-dimensional strategy for Leadership is suggested (i) Initiatives appealing (ii) Integrating all (iii) Incremental advancements. The 'Five Es' for Teamwork, and the 'Five Cs' for Organizational Change are elaborated. Artificial Intelligence has the potential to improve healthcare safety. AI enables analysis of data from multiple sources simultaneously using advanced algorithms. This identifies predictors and outcomes. Ensemble learning algorithms, used by advanced practitioners of machine learning, are useful with high final accuracy. Hence in matters of health these should be utilized. All this will make prevention targeted, better, and timely.

Keywords: errors, side effects, hospital design, nosocomial, stress ulcers, pneumonia, management, artificial intelligence, algorithms, prediction

1. Introduction

"To err is human & not to err is not a hype, but an achievable ability"

Delivering the right care at the right time in the right setting is the core mission of Hospitals. Hospitalization has its inherent complications and medical errors can further compromise patient safety. Institute of Medicine's sentinel report "To Err is Human: Building a Safer Health System" is a worldwide inspiration wonderful [1]. The report advanced patient safety and stimulated dedicated research funding to this essential aspect of patient care. Since then, highly effective interventions have been developed and adopted for hospital-acquired infections and medication safety [2]. Progress and perfection in addressing other hospital adverse events is desirable.

Medical errors are a serious public health problem. Patient safety is fundamental to high-quality patient care. Preventive strategies for patient safety are the need of the hour.

Hospitals provides an opportunity for practicing preventive medicine. Two important areas are (i) to make treatment and hospitalization free from side-effects (like bed rest/immobility complications, nosocomial infections, treatment side-effects, etc) (ii) obviate medical errors. Although the scope of preventive medicine in hospitals is wide, we need to focus on important issues on priority.

There is growing awareness of the frequency, causes, and consequences of errors as well as side effects in medicine, all for progress for perfection. All this makes it important that we devise workable solutions – the prevention strategies.

"Trying to ensure the safest possible patient care is
as old as medicine itself"
'Primum non nocere' (First, do no harm) is
one of the core principles of medical practice.

1.1 Why hospitals?

Hospitals should be on the top of priority list. This is because medical errors may occur in different health care settings, and those that happen in hospitals can have serious consequences [3]. Health care organizations are struggling universally to identify and remediate safety-related challenges.

2. Methodical paradigm

Threats to patient safety result from complex causes. Improvements for safety are possible with analysis of causes of error. With this knowledge we need to design '*Preventive systems of care*' so as to make errors less common and less harmful when they do occur" [4].

The steps for practice of preventive Medicine in Hospitals should be

i. Intervention design: Defining and designing the content and the implementation plan of the intervention

ii. Intervention implementation

iii. Intervention institutionalization

2.1 Defining the problem

Critical steps toward improving the safety of the health care system include ensuring that the system is aware of what errors can occur and thus leading to formulation of effective remedies – Preventive action plan.

Internationally, an important study in this regard has been *The Harvard Medical Practice Study*. This was an interdisciplinary study of medical injury and malpractice, and was conducted in the early 1990s [5].

The first part of this study focused on the incidence of adverse events, defined as injuries resulting from negligent or substandard care. *Brennan et al.* reported that adverse events occurred in 3.7 percent of the hospitalizations (95% confidence interval [CI] = 3.2–4.2). Also, they reported that 27.6 percent (95% CI = 22.5–32.6) of the adverse events were due to negligence. Further, 13.6 percent of the adverse events led to the death of the patient [5].

The second part of the Harvard Medical Practice Study analyzed the records of 1,133 patients who had disabling injuries caused by medical treatment. *Brennan et al.* reported that among these patients, drug complications were the most common type of adverse event (19 percent), followed by wound infections (14 percent) and technical complications (13 percent) [6].

The latest figures are still disturbing. Patient harm due to adverse events is one of the top 10 causes of death and disability in the world [7].

2.2 Prevention strategies: concepts

Modern health care is highly complex, high risk, and error prone. All this makes, not surprisingly, health care errors and consequent adverse events a leading cause of death and injury. Well-documented methods to prevent the occurrence of many of these errors need to be constantly evolved. Safe Practices reducing the risk of harm resulting from the processes, systems, or environments of care are required. Patient safety should be the highest priority for health care providers [8].

2.3 Prevention strategies: environment

2.3.1 Hospital design

> *"We shape our buildings and afterwards our buildings shape us."*
> *Winston Churchill*

Evidence-based design is a term used to describe how the physical design of health care environments affects patients and staff [9]. Key characteristics of evidence-based design in hospital settings include single-patient rooms, use of noise-reducing construction materials, easily accessible workstations, and improved layout for patients and staff [10].

Several scholars highlighted that Evidence based design for built environment can lower the incidence of nosocomial infections, medical errors, patient falls, and staff injuries [11]. Patient safety can be enhanced through flexibility and adaptability. The following need to be ensured:

1. Ensuring adequate space for work areas improves patient and staff outcomes [12]. More space for staff to provide care ensures safety. Less space more errors likely. More space can accommodate new, advanced procedures and diagnostics.

2. The windows of patient rooms should be adequately sized. Purposes served are improving visibility of patients for monitoring and also providing view of natural surroundings. Monitoring adequate ensures early safety energetically, mitigating errors or side-effects if any.

3. Light sources within rooms mimic natural light, promoting natural feelings, rather than exaggerating adverse feelings associated with hospitalization [13].

2.3.2 Art in art and science of medicine & patient safety perspective

Hospital environment should be pleasing, and art is an added advantage. Hospitalization is stressful, and stress can lead to multiplied side-effect of hospitalization, hence needs to be relieved. Artwork may enhance the effects on patient satisfaction, feeling of self-control and distraction by attractive stimuli. Art has positive effects on well-being and behavior. Natural scenes in patient rooms and diverse art in public areas should be preferred [14]. All this will alleviate the likely problems patients may face.

White coat hypertension needs attention, and recent evidence shows it is not innocent [15]. A Randomized Controlled Trial has shown that landscape photographic art in medical office examination rooms may have the beneficial effect of reducing white coat hypertension. The results show statistically significant difference between the mean arterial pressure, systolic BP and diastolic BP between the control room and the photo room [16].

2.4 Settings and strategies

2.4.1 Intensive Care Units (ICU)

Prevention of Complications of Critical Illness in ICU is important.

a. Venous thromboembolism (VTE)

This is a serious complication for patients in the intensive care unit (ICU) [17]. All ICU patients are at high risk for this complication given their predilection toward immobility. It includes upper and lower extremity deep vein thrombosis (DVT) and pulmonary embolism (PE). Therefore, all ICU patients should receive some form of prophylaxis against VTE.

A recent Systematic review and network meta-analysis of randomized clinical trials (RCTs) has concluded that LMWH reduces incidence of DVT, while UFH and mechanical compressive devices may reduce the risk of DVT. LMWH is probably more effective than UFH in reducing incidence of DVT. It should be considered the primary pharmacologic agent for thromboprophylaxis. The efficacy and safety of combination pharmacologic therapy and mechanical compressive devices is unclear [18].

b. Stress ulcers

Currently available data suggest that high-risk patients, such as those with coagulopathy, shock, or respiratory failure requiring mechanical ventilation, benefit from prophylactic treatment.
Prophylaxis against stress ulcers is frequently administered in most ICUs. Typically, histamine-2 antagonists are administered, and are preferred over proton pump inhibitors.

c. Prevention of pneumonia

Intensive care unit (ICU) acquired pneumonia is amongst the most common and morbid health care-associated infections.
Interventions reducing length of ICU stay reduces pneumonia incidence and should be prioritized. Other effective strategies are avoiding intubation, minimizing sedation, implementing early extubation strategies, and mobilizing patients. Dramatic decreases in Ventilator Associated Pneumonia rates occurs with implementation of ventilator bundles (**Table 1**). Best practices for implementation are engaging and educating staff and creating structures that facilitate bundle adherence. Regular feedback on process measure performance and outcome rates leads to improvements [19, 20].

2.4.2 Nosocomial infections

25–50% or more of nosocomial infections are due to the combined effect of the patient's own flora and invasive devices. There is a need for improvements in the use of such devices. Intensive education and "bundling" of evidence-based interventions (**Table 1**) can reduce infection rates through improved asepsis in handling and earlier removal of invasive devices. The maintenance of such gains requires ongoing efforts.

2.4.3 Neonatal ICU

Nosocomial infections are among the leading causes of mortality and morbidity in neonatal intensive care units.

Preventive strategies are (i) hand hygiene practices (ii) central venous (CVC)-related bloodstream infections prevention (iii) judicious use of antimicrobials for therapy (iv) enhancement of host defences with early enteral feeding with human milk (v) skin care.

2.4.4 Surgical safety

Adverse events have been estimated to affect 3–16% of all hospitalized patients. Surgical care contributes to half of these. More than half of such events are preventable [21].

One must be open to learning, embracing, and perfecting new surgical techniques of proven value. These include minimal tissue trauma, short operation times with brief ischemia periods, minimal blood loss etc [22]. Surgical progress with microsurgical techniques is leading the way for precision, perfection, and fewer complications [23].

Surgery has become more complex with more sophisticated technology and patients with more diverse and complex co-morbidities are being operated. Multiple

Central Venous Catheter Infections	*Catheter insertion*	• Training of personnel about catheter insertion and care. • Chlorhexidine for insertion site preparation. • Maximal barrier precautions and asepsis during catheter insertion. • Insertion supplies consolidation (e.g., in an insertion kit or cart). • Checklist to enhance adherence to the insertion bundle. • Halt insertion if asepsis is breached.
	Catheter maintenance	• Cleansing daily with chlorhexidine. • Clean & dry dressings. • Hand hygiene maintenance of health care workers.
	Daily assessment of need of the catheter. Remove catheter if not needed or used.	
Prevention of Ventilator-Associated Events	• Mechanical ventilation use only when absolutely necessary. • Elevation of head of bed to 30–45° • "Sedation vacation": a balancing act of tightly titrating the sedative dose to provide agitation free, comfortable sedation on the lowest dosage possible • Assessment for readiness to extubate daily. • Deep-vein thrombosis prophylaxis (unless contraindicated).	
Prevention of Surgical-Site Infections	• Right surgeon for right surgery. • Prophylactic antibiotics within 1 h before surgery; discontinuation within 24 h. • Limit any hair removal to the time of surgery; use clippers or do not remove hair at all. • Surgical site preparation with chlorhexidine-alcohol.	
Prevention of Urinary Tract Infections	• Bladder catheters use only when absolutely needed (e.g., to relieve obstruction). • Aseptic equipment and technique for catheter insertion and urinary tract instrumentation. • Manipulation or opening of drainage systems minimized. • Daily assessment of bladder catheter need? Remove if not needed.	
Prevention of Pathogen Cross-Transmission	• Hands cleansing with alcohol hand rub before and after all contacts with patients or their environments.	

Adapted from: www.cdc.gov/hicpac/pubs.html; www.cdc.gov/HAI/index.html.

Table 1.
Evidence based "Bundled Interventions" to prevent common health care–associated infections and other adverse events.

team surgeries from diverse sub-specialties are becoming more common. These also entail risk of more errors. Dr. Atul Gawande, Professor of Surgery at Harvard Medical School, argues that using checklists can help surgeons to cope with increasing complexity. Use of a rigorous checklist in this rapidly changing environment will consolidate surgeons' aims to enhance both patient safety and clinical professionalism [24].

Strategy for wrong-site, wrong-patient, wrong-procedure events

Although, such events are rare but the consequences can be devastating. Hence prevention is of utmost importance.

Recent efforts made to address and prevent wrong-site surgery by a team at Naval Hospital, Cherry Point, NC (NHCP), have exemplified this [25]. Surgical verification checklist and its implementation provides for quality, safety, and a commitment to patient care.

2.4.5 Maternal and newborn health

While in most cases having a baby is a positive experience, pregnancy and childbirth can cause suffering, ill health or even death. Every year, women and newborn babies die from complications related to childbirth.

The interventions and approaches that help save the lives of mothers and babies are well documented (**Table 2**). They can work even where resources are poor [26].

Maternal hospital care	• Hygiene and accident prevention (staff) Staff has access to fully equipped hand washing facilities. Sharps are disposed of in a special container to prevent accidents • Hygienic conditions (mothers) There are sufficient and adequate toilets which are clean and easily accessible. Mothers have access to running water, soap and to an appropriate space, near the ward, to wash themselves and their child. Mothers have access to a washing facility for washing theirs and their babies' clothes. • Rooming in Newborn babies are roomed in with their mothers. Proper place for changing diapers of their babies. • Attention for the most seriously ill women These should be cared for in a section where they receive closer attention - close to the nursing station (can be directly observed most of the time).
Nursery	• Separate room for sick newborn babies Mothers of these are allowed to stay with their babies • Hygienic services for mothers Toilets are adequate and easily available Mothers have access to running water and to an appropriate space, near the ward to wash themselves and their child • Special attention for the most seriously ill newborn babies The most seriously ill infants are cared for in a section near the nursing station for direct observation

Table 2.
Quality mother and newborn care features and facilities.

2.4.6 Hospital laboratories

Medical laboratory test data is increasingly being utilized. Medical laboratory should provide the doctor and the patient accurate, precise, and reliable results. Medical test malpractice can lead to a medical accident. Hence the need of quality and safety assurance with management of the overall processes required to provide high quality medical laboratory results [27]. Results should be transcribed in a reliable way and all necessary information should be provided for the correct interpretation of results [28]. It needs to be ensured that critical and alarming results are communicated to clinicians immediately.

2.4.7 Transitions in care – handing over

In health care organizations patients are subjected to multiple transitions in care. This is inevitable as continuous, 24-hour treatment necessitates the division of labor [29]. These transitions, or "handovers," are potential points of failure, thus making preventive actions of utmost important. Gaps in handover communication between patient care units, and between and among care teams, can cause serious breakdowns in the continuity of care, inappropriate treatment, and potential harm for the patient. Proper handing over of all information and spending time on this is the best preventive solution.

2.4.8 Radiation risks minimization

Radiological investigation should be ordered after clinical impact assessment by clinicians. These should be individually tailored by the radiologist using the least parameters of exposure. Paediatric patients vulnerability justifies special attention [30].

Radiation therapy acute toxicities can be alleviated by giving gap in the treatment. Chronic toxicities are more serious. Overall clinical outcomes of radiotherapy are optimized when radiotherapy services function along with effective prevention, early detection programs, and quality surgery [30].

2.4.9 Special clinics

Comprehensive treatment in the outpatient setting, including of patients with complex disorders is possible in Special Clinics. This needs encouragement. This has cost advantages as well as reduces the adverse side-effects of hospital stays [31]. Establishing an asthma clinic has been demonstrated to decrease hospitalizations [32].

3. Managerial perspectives

Hospital governance is increasingly encompassing 'improving performance on clinical outcomes'. Coordination of medicine and management across the levels of hospital/department is for quality-effective hospital governance [33]. The managers themselves seem to rely more on personal strength and medical knowledge than on management tools [34]. Medical expertise benefits management evidently. Doctors are increasingly involved in hospital management. This is likely to lead to better implemented quality management systems [35].

Among physicians, there is a growing sense of the responsibility as teachers of better habits of life and work, and hospitals in like manner are becoming more truly educational centers in preventive medicine [36]. Prevention for safety needs to be practiced by all.

3.1 Money matters

It has been shown that patients treated at financially distressed hospitals are more likely to have adverse patient safety events [37]. This suggests that hospitals should be financially sound, ensuring safety of patients. Cost-cutting efforts should be carefully designed and managed, without compromising quality and safety.

3.2 Leadership

With evolution of safety field, there is a growing recognition that organizational leadership plays a role in prioritizing safety [38]. Hospital boards have an important role of in overseeing patient quality and safety. It has been shown that high-performing hospitals have board members who were more skilled in quality and safety issues and who devoted more time to discussion of quality and safety [39]. Patient safety performance by hospitals adds to good reputation.

We suggest three-dimensional initiatives for Leaders:

i. **Initiatives appealing**: Strategic initiatives are required for quality and safety. Written policies for pertinent workability should be in place. Frequent trainings should be organized.

ii. **Integrating all**: Actions at the ground level should be safe and sound. Leaders should visit clinical units, interact with workers, discuss concerns and provide solutions. Motivation will ensure quality and safety.

iii. **Incremental advancements**: rewards for good results and opposite for the contrary, are required. Leaders should ensure unprofessional or incompetent clinicians do not put patients at risk [38]. Increments for good performance and early intervention for unprofessional behavior by hospital leadership will set the pace for excellence.

3.3 Teamwork – a blueprint

Teamwork is a powerful patient safety tool. The U.S. Department of Defense (DoD) Military Health System provided essential insight for Teamwork development [40]. Teamwork initiatives are effective with a clear blueprint defining the solid steps for building the desired culture. Characteristics for success of the blueprint are clear, detailed, and self-evident. All this should include the 'Five Es'

i. Establish vision of, and for, teams

ii. Environment planning and preparation

iii. Expectations and behaviours training for implementation

iv. Expertly monitor and coach to sustain behaviors

v. Energetically align and integrate the behaviors [40].

3.4 Organizational change for patient safety initiatives

Patient safety accomplishment requires not only clinical efforts but also organizational. Widespread organizational change for betterment in patient safety is indispensable. The implementation of patient safety initiatives should be done utilizing change management principles, namely the 'Five Cs'

i. Congruent changes targeting multiple components

ii. Change management roles specific for different participants in the care-delivery process

iii. Concrete implementation through dedicated support structures and multiple tactics

iv. Complete institutionalization through enhanced workforce capabilities

v. Continuous learning and improvements [41, 42].

3.5 Science to Service: tailor made solutions

Progressive evidence on patient safety is increasingly available, and refines practices. The eventual users of these are many and diverse, including administrators and managers, and health care professionals, such as physicians, nurses, pharmacists and laboratory technicians. Research findings and applications of these should be tailor made for different groups for implementation [43].

3.6 Sophisticated management simplified

- Avenues and attitudes: Identification of problematic areas and orientation in attitudes of the workforce

- Betterment and beautification: Building on strengths and beautification for ubiquitous success

- Comprehensive with conviction: All aspects need to be considered involving everyone with conviction to act and achieve

- Diligence for making a difference: Meticulous efforts for scrupulous results

- Energized for excellence: It requires sustained energy leading to excellence, to achieve the targets, and to stay high on the results [44].

4. Artificial Intelligence advancements

A person working in partnership with an information resource is "better" than that same person unassisted. This is the "Fundamental Theorem" of Biomedical Informatics [45]. Computer Science is making rapid progress and affecting all aspects of human activities. Artificial intelligence (AI) is an interesting domain. It utilizes computers and technology to simulate intelligent behavior and critical thinking comparable to a human being. Its applications for patient safety need to be explored.

The increasing availability of data and emerging technologies needs to be best converged and utilized for better healthcare. A conceptual framework for this leading to AI Patient Safety applications is proposed (**Figure 1**). The AI applications are broadly classified into five categories:

1. AI for proper assessment

2. AI for pertinent treatment

3. AI for progress monitoring

4. AI for prevention applications

5. AI for professional standards

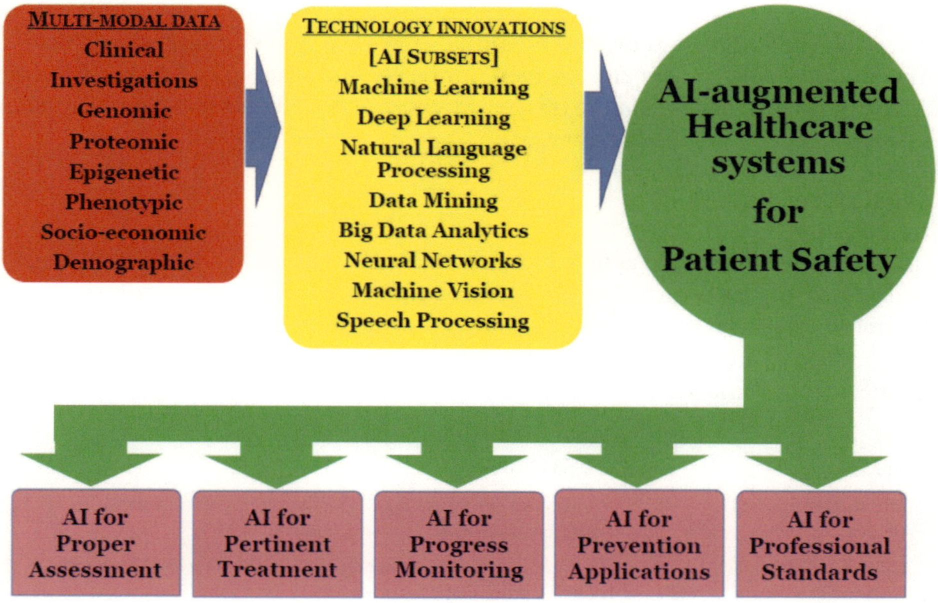

Figure 1.
Conceptual framework for AI patient safety applications.

4.1 AI for proper assessment

Clinical assessment involves history taking, clinical examination, investigations leading to diagnosis. Diagnostic error as an area of patient safety has had insufficient research in spite of the negative health outcomes it can lead to [1]. Evidence is accumulating that computer-based trigger algorithms may reduce delayed diagnosis and improve diagnostic accuracy [46].

4.1.1 Future progress

Diagnostic error causation is very complex and typically occur from the convergence of multiple contributing factors [47]. Lack of medical data can lead to inefficient or inappropriate practice [48]. There are opportunities for improvement using Electronic Health Record (EHR) data sources and AI. ML could help to reduce the frequency of diagnostic errors by improving upon limitation factors of clinicians, namely pattern recognition, bias, and limited capacity [49].

The focus should be on the 'Big Three diseases' which account for about three-fourths of serious misdiagnosis-related harms, namely vascular events, infections, and cancers [50].

4.2 AI for pertinent treatment

Selecting right medications, rightly planned surgeries, right counselling are all benefitted by technology, ensuring patient safety.

Computer-generated prescriptions have many benefits, including links to software that highlights risks from drugs or drug-drug combinations [51]. AI can lead to further improvements and alerts for mistakes.

3D printing is enabling precision surgery. Virtual surgical planning using information regarding patient anatomy and medical devices to be used in surgery increase confidence and knowledge before surgery for better outcomes [52]. Further AI applications can be built with real time image processing capabilities which alert surgeons of any deviations from precision surgery.

4.2.1 Future progress

AI can analysis vast data at lightening fast speed. All EHRs need to be analysed for side-effects of medicines, including correlation with the doses prescribed. Refinements are always needed to minimize side-effects [53].

AI for correct prescriptions should first focus on medications that commonly result in errors (**Table 3**).

Medication	Mechanisms
Antithrombotic agents	Insufficient dosing leading to a thrombotic event like a stroke, excess dosing resulting in bleeding
Cardioplegic solutions	Errors in preparation, team breakdown, lack of technical competence, and poor monitoring of the patient
Chemotherapeutic agents	Administering the wrong dose, wrong drug, wrong number of days supplied, and missed doses). In addition, drug administration errors including wrong flow rate or failure to monitor the site of intravenous (IV) transfusion are often reported with chemotherapeutic drugs administered intravenously.
Dialysis solutions	Administering the wrong medication, wrong dose, infection at the site, hyperkalemia, patient falls, and access-related errors
Epidural or intrathecal medications	Erroneous infusions-administering an IV medication via the intrathecal route, giving wrong medication or wrong dose
Hypertonic solutions	Failure to monitor for renal failure, edema, hyperchloremic metabolic acidosis, coagulation abnormalities
Hypertonic sodium chloride for injection	Failure to monitor for renal failure, confusion, coma, seizures
Hypoglycemic agents	Failure to do dose adjustment with monitoring for hypoglycemic episodes

Adapted from reference Rodziewicz et al. [47].

Table 3.
Medications commonly resulting in errors.

4.3 AI for progress monitoring

Monitoring is required, useful, and remotely done is advantageous. Technology is useful for all this. Fast data transmission for favourable timely actions is the ultimate aim. AI can make all this expertly efficient.

4.3.1 Future progress

The advancements of biomedical sensing and healthcare information technology have resulted in data-rich environments in hospitals. Analysis of all this data for actionable in sights is possible with AI. AI systems need to be developed for real time fast alerts to mitigate crisis leading to increased patient safety. The shortage of doctors, long duty hours for monitoring, right doctors for right patients etc will be all benefited.

4.4 AI for prevention applications

Clinical deterioration in the hospital is common and has to be energetically assessed and prevented.

ICU treatment involves multitude of data, both clinical and laboratory investigations. The Pediatric Logistic Organ Dysfunction (PELOD) score is based on the relative severities among Organ Dysfunctions (ODs) and the degree of severity of each OD using logistic regression [54]. A machine learning model, using random forest classifier, has achieved better performance than this [55]. Ensemble learning algorithms, used by advanced practitioners of machine learning, are useful with high final accuracy. Hence in matters of health these should be utilized.

4.4.1 Future progress

Future work should focus on inferring and predicting based on new categories of data, including biometric sensors like continuous telemetry, motion activity sensors, novel biomarkers, and relevant patient-reported measures [49].

4.5 AI for professional standards

Excellence & competency ensures correct treatment, free from errors and side effects. AI augmentation of human performance is likely to be of widespread use [56]. AI technology can provide decision support to clinicians seeking to find the best diagnosis and treatment for patients [57]. This coupled with doctor's competence should lead to professional standards and patient safety of highest order.

4.5.1 Future progress

Systematic analysis for sophisticated advancements is regularly required [58]. Machine Learning has capabilities of reading, processing, and interpreting the available data (structured and unstructured) at enormous scale and volume. New evidence can be synthesized, all for patient treatment perfect.

New evidence is accumulating at a fast pace. It is difficult for doctors to keep pace. Systematic Reviews and Meta-Analysis requires humongous efforts. AI applications can be developed for automated Systematic Reviews and Meta-Analysis. Concise results of these will be useful for all. Progress features promise exciting future [59].

AI has the potential to revolutionize the teaching and practice of Surgery. The ways for this are (i) AI analysis of population and patient-specific data for improvements in each phase of surgical care (iii) AI enabling and making easy access of surgical experience repositories for sharing of knowledge. This includes collection of massive amounts of operative video and EMR data across many surgeons. This will lead to a future optimized for the highest quality patient care [56].

5. Conclusion

Patient safety is always required and ensures high-quality patient care. The inherent complications of hospitalization can be prevented with strategies suggested. Medical errors diverse causation needs high alert for all factors. Our suggested preventive strategies will ensure excellence. Managerial expertise is required for high standards for patient safety. Artificial Intelligence has the potential to improve healthcare safety. AI applications will make prevention targeted, better, and timely.

> *"Clinical excellence, Management methodical, &*
> *Artificial Intelligence advancements,*
> *All for safe and sound patient outcomes perfect"*

Acknowledgements

Thankful to the authors and publishers of all the references quoted.

Conflict of interest

The authors declare no conflict of interest.

Author details

Sunil Jain[1*], Bhagya Kamal Jain[2], Prem Kamal Jain[3] and Arvind Singh Kushwaha[4]

1 Department of Paediatrics, Military Hospital Secunderabad, Telangana State, India

2 Google Inc., India

3 Department of Computational Biology, Indraprastha Institute of Information Technology, New Delhi, India

4 All India Institute of Medical Sciences, Nagpur, India

*Address all correspondence to: sunil_jain700@rediff.com

References

[1] Institute of Medicine (US) Committee on Quality of Health Care in America. In: Kohn LT, Corrigan JM, Donaldson MS, editors. To Err is Human: Building a Safer Health System. Washington (DC): National Academies Press (US); 2000

[2] Bates DW, Singh H. Two decades since to err is human: An assessment of progress and emerging priorities in patient safety. Health Affiliation (Millwood). 2018;**37**(11):1736-1743

[3] 10 Patient Safety Tips for Hospitals. The Agency for Healthcare Research and Quality. Available from: http://www.ahrq.gov; https://www.ahrq.gov/patients-consumers/diagnosis-treatment/hospitals-clinics/10-tips/index.html [Accessed June 16, 2022]

[4] Stone PW, Harrison MI, Feldman P, et al. Organizational climate of staff working conditions and safety—An integrative model. In: Henriksen K, Battles JB, Marks ES, et al., editors. Advances in Patient Safety: From Research to Implementation. Rockville (MD): Agency for Healthcare Research and Quality (US); 2005

[5] Brennan TA, Leape LL, Laird NM, et al. Incidence of adverse events and negligence in hospitalized patients. Results of the Harvard Medical Practice Study I. New England Journal of Medicine. 1991;**324**(6):370-376

[6] Brennan TA, Leape LL, Laird NM, et al. The nature of adverse events in hospitalized patients. Results of the Harvard Medical Practice Study II. The New England Journal of Medicine. 1991;**324**(6):377-384

[7] "Patient Safety - A Grand Challenge for Healthcare Professionals and Policymakers Alike" a Roundtable at the Grand Challenges Meeting of the Bill & Melinda Gates Foundation, 18 October 2018. Available from: https://globalhealth.harvard.edu/qualitypowerpoint [Accessed June 15, 2022]

[8] Clair JS. A new model of tracheostomy care: Closing the research–practice gap. In: Henriksen K, Battles JB, Marks ES, et al., editors. Advances in Patient Safety: From Research to Implementation. Rockville (MD): Agency for Healthcare Research and Quality (US); 2005

[9] Kirk HD. Evidence-based practice: Four levels revisited. HERD. 2020;**13**(3):26-29

[10] The Center for Health Design. Scorecards for Evidence-Based Design. Concord, CA; 2005

[11] Ulrich RS, Berry LL, Quan X, Parish JT. A conceptual framework for the domain of evidence-based design. HERD. 2010;**4**(1):95-114

[12] Reiling J, Hughes RG, Murphy MR. The impact of facility design on patient safety. In: Hughes RG, editor. Patient Safety and Quality: An Evidence-Based Handbook for Nurses. Rockville (MD): Agency for Healthcare Research and Quality (US); 2008

[13] Reiling JG. Creating a Culture of Patient Safety through Innovative Hospital Design. In: Henriksen K, Battles JB, Marks ES, et al., editors. Advances in Patient Safety: From Research to Implementation. Rockville (MD): Agency for Healthcare Research and Quality (US); 2005

[14] Fudickar A, Konetzka D, Nielsen SML, Hathorn K. Evidence-based

art in the hospital. Wiener Medizinische Wochenschrift (1946). 2022;**172**(9-10):234-241. DOI: 10.1007/s10354-021-00861-7

[15] Mancia G, Facchetti R, Bombelli M, Cuspidi C, Grassi G. White-coat hypertension: Pathophysiological and clinical aspects: Excellence Award for Hypertension Research 2020. Hypertension. 2021;**78**(6):1677-1688

[16] Harper MB, Kanayama-Trivedi S, Caldito G, Montgomery D, Mayeaux EJ Jr, DelRosso LM. Photographic art in exam rooms may reduce white coat hypertension. Medical Humanities. 2015;**41**(2):86-88

[17] Geerts WH, Bergqvist D, Pineo GF, et al. Prevention of venous thromboembolism: American College of Chest Physicians Evidence-Based Clinical Practice Guidelines (8th Edition). Chest. 2008;**133**(6):381-453

[18] Fernando SM, Tran A, Cheng W, et al. VTE prophylaxis in critically ill adults: A systematic review and network meta-analysis. Chest. 2022;**161**(2):418-428

[19] Klompas M. Prevention of intensive care unit-acquired pneumonia. Seminars in Respiratory and Critical Care Medicine. 2019;**40**(4):548-557

[20] Klompas M. What is new in the prevention of nosocomial pneumonia in the ICU? Current Opinion in Critical Care. 2017;**23**(5):378-384

[21] WHO Guidelines for Safe Surgery: Safe Surgery Saves Lives. 2009. Available from: https://www.who.int/publications/i/item/9789241598552 [Accessed June 15, 2022]

[22] Vuille-Dit-Bille RN. Special issue on surgical innovation: New surgical devices, techniques, and progress in surgical training. The Journal of International Medical Research. 2020;**48**(3):300

[23] Jain S. Congenital heart disease: Saving lives and securing liveliness with early primary care and expert family care. Journal of Family Medicine and Primary Care. 2021;**10**(9):3178-3184

[24] Gawande A. The Checklist Manifesto: How to Do Things Right. New York: Henry Holt and Company; 2009

[25] Ludwick S. Surgical safety: addressing the JCAHO goals for reducing wrong-site, wrong-patient, wrong-procedure events. In: Henriksen K, Battles JB, Marks ES, et al., editors. Advances in Patient Safety: From Research to Implementation. Rockville (MD): Agency for Healthcare Research and Quality (US); 2005

[26] MAKING PREGNANCY SAFER Assessment tool for the quality of hospital care for mothers and newborn babies. World Health Organization Regional Office for Europe. Available from: http://www.euro.who.int/pubrequest [Accessed June 1, 2022]

[27] Kayamori Y, Fujishima A, Noda N, et al. Approach for prevention of medical test malpractice using ISO 15189. Rinsho Byori. 2010;**58**(8):839-846

[28] Yeste MLL, Álvarez SI. Management of postanalytical processes in the clinical laboratory according to ISO 15189:2012 Standard requirements: considerations on the review, reporting and release of results. Advances in Laboratory Medicine / Avances en Medicina de Laboratorio. 2021;**2**(1):51-59

[29] Behara R, Wears RL, Perry SJ, et al. Conceptual Framework for Studying the Safety of Transitions in Emergency Care.

In: Henriksen K, Battles JB, Marks ES, Lewin DI, editors. Advances in Patient Safety: From Research to Implementation. Rockville (MD): Agency for Healthcare Research and Quality (US); 2005

[30] Jain S. Radiation in medical practice & health effects of radiation: Rationale, risks, and rewards. Journal of Family Medicine and Primary Care. 2021;**10**(4):1520-1524

[31] Jain S, Dewey RS. The role of "Special Clinics" in imparting clinical skills: Medical education for competence and sophistication. Advances in Medical Education and Practice. 2021;**12**:513-518

[32] Jain S, Thapar RK, Mallick A, Tiwari S, Yokesh D, Abhijit YV. Evidence based focused approach for fulfillment of aims: Experiences of an asthma clinic. Indian Journal of Child Health. 2017;**4**:170-175

[33] Kuhlmann E, Burau V, Correia T, Lewandowski R, Lionis C, Noordegraaf M, et al. "A manager in the minds of doctors:" a comparison of new modes of control in European hospitals. BMC Health Services Research. 2013;**13**:246. DOI: 10.1186/1472-6963-13-246

[34] Kuhlmann E, Rangnitt Y, von Knorring M. Medicine and management: looking inside the box of changing hospital governance. BMC Health Services Research. 2016;**16**:159

[35] Rotar AM, Botje D, Klazinga NS, et al. The involvement of medical doctors in hospital governance and implications for quality management: a quick scan in 19 and an in depth study in 7 OECD countries. BMC Health Services Research. 2016;**16**:160

[36] Wright W. The hospital and industrial hygiene. American Journal of Public Health (N Y). 1917;**7**(11):949-952. DOI: 10.2105/ajph.7.11.949

[37] Bernard D, Encinosa WE. Financial and Demographic Influences on Medicare Patient Safety Events. In: Henriksen K, Battles JB, Marks ES, et al., editors. Advances in Patient Safety: From Research to Implementation. Rockville (MD): Agency for Healthcare Research and Quality (US); 2005

[38] Patient Safety Network (PSNet) Leadership Role in Improving Safety. Available from: https://psnet.ahrq.gov/primer/leadership-role-improving-safety [Accessed June 16, 2022]

[39] Millar R, Mannion R, Freeman T, Davies HT. Hospital board oversight of quality and patient safety: a narrative review and synthesis of recent empirical research. The Milbank Quarterly. 2013;**91**(4):738-770. DOI: 10.1111/1468-0009.12032

[40] King HB, Kohsin B, Salisbury M. Systemwide deployment of medical team training: lessons learned in the department of defense. In: Henriksen K, Battles JB, Marks ES, et al., editors. Advances in Patient Safety: From Research to Implementation. Rockville (MD): Agency for Healthcare Research and Quality (US); 2005

[41] Ramanujam R, Keyser DJ, Sirio CA. Making a case for organizational change in patient safety initiatives. In: Henriksen K, Battles JB, Marks ES, et al., editors. Advances in Patient Safety: From Research to Implementation. Rockville (MD): Agency for Healthcare Research and Quality (US); 2005

[42] Anderson JG, Ramanujam R, Hensel D, Anderson MM, Sirio CA. The need for organizational change in patient safety initiatives. International Journal of Medical Informatics. Dec 2006;**75**(12):809-817

[43] Nieva VF, Murphy R, Ridley N, et al. From science to service: A framework for the transfer of patient safety research into practice. In: Henriksen K, Battles JB, Marks ES, et al., editors. Advances in Patient Safety: From Research to Implementation. Rockville (MD): Agency for Healthcare Research and Quality (US); 2005

[44] Jain S, Thapar RK. Hygiene & health: effects, experiences & expertise of 'Clean India Campaign' from a Tertiary Care Hospital. Indian Journal of Child Health. 2017;**4**(4):518-522

[45] Friedman CP. A "fundamental theorem" of biomedical informatics. Journal of the American Medical Informatics Association. 2009;**16**(2):169-170. DOI: 10.1197/jamia.M3092

[46] Abimanyi-Ochom J, Bohingamu Mudiyanselage S, Catchpool M, et al. Strategies to reduce diagnostic errors: a systematic review. BMC Medical Informatics and Decision Making. 2019;**19**(1):174. DOI: 10.1186/s12911-019-0901-1

[47] Rodziewicz TL, Houseman B, Hipskind JE. Medical Error Reduction and Prevention. Treasure Island (FL): StatPearls Publishing; 2022

[48] Lieutenant Colonel Sunil Jain, MD. The Smart Indian Soldier. Journal of the United Service Institution of India. 2011;**CXLI**(583):101-109. Available from: https://usiofindia.org/publication/usi-journal/the-smart-indian-soldier

[49] Bates DW, Levine D, Syrowatka A, Kuznetsova M, Craig KJT, Rui A, et al. The potential of artificial intelligence to improve patient safety: a scoping review. NPJ Digital Medicine. 2021;**4**(1):54. DOI: 10.1038/s41746-021-00423-6

[50] Newman-Toker DE, Schaffer AC, Yu-Moe CW, et al. Serious misdiagnosis-related harms in malpractice claims: The "Big Three" – vascular events, infections, and cancers. Diagnosis (Berl). 2019;**6**(3):227

[51] Trent RJ. Omics. In: Trent RJ, editor. Molecular Medicine, Fourth Edition. London: Academic Press; 2012. pp. 117-152. ISBN: 9780123814517. DOI: 10.1016/B978-0-12-381451-7.00004-9

[52] Chepelev L, Wake N, Ryan J, et al. RSNA Special Interest Group for 3D Printing. Radiological Society of North America (RSNA) 3D printing Special Interest Group (SIG): guidelines for medical 3D printing and appropriateness for clinical scenarios. 3D Print Medicine. 2018;**4**(1):11

[53] Jain S, Santhosh A. Febrile seizures: Evidence for evolution of an operational strategy from an Armed Forces referral hospital. Pediatric Health, Medicine and Therapeutics. 2021;**12**:151-159

[54] Leteurtre S, Martinot A, Duhamel A, Gauvin F, Grandbastien B, Nam TV, et al. Development of a pediatric multiple organ dysfunction score: use of two strategies. Medical Decision Making. 1999;**19**(4):399-410

[55] Prince RD, Akhondi-Asl A, Mehta NM, Geva A. A Machine learning classifier improves mortality prediction compared with pediatric logistic organ dysfunction-2 score: Model development and validation. Crit Care Exploration. 2021;**3**(5):e0426

[56] Hashimoto DA, Rosman G, Rus D, Meireles OR. Artificial intelligence in surgery: Promises and Perils. Annals of Surgery. 2018;**268**(1):70-76. DOI: 10.1097/SLA.0000000000002693

[57] Davenport T, Kalakota R. The potential for artificial intelligence in

healthcare. Future Healthcare Journal. 2019;**6**(2):94-98. DOI: 10.7861/futurehosp.6-2-94

[58] Jain S, Chandra N, Thapar RK. Paediatric Surgery experiences of a tertiary referral hospital: International Classification of Diseases Spectrum for teaching, planning, & scaling up services. Indian Journal of Child Health. 2019;**6**(6):313-319

[59] Jain S. Clinico-pathological correlation: Teaching aspects, avenues, & advances. Journal of Advances in Medical Education & Professionalism. 2022;**10**(1):59-63

Chapter 11

Clinical Futile Cycles: Systematic Microeconomic Reform of Health Care by Reform of the Traditional Hierarchical Referral Model of Care

Michael Buist and Georgia Arnold

Abstract

The incidence of adverse patient events in hospitals has not improved over the last two decades despite enormous efforts in the area of Quality and Safety. Notably, the same errors are often repeated, even though previous reviews of these events have resulted in learnings, guidelines and policy. The traditional review of a Hospital Adverse Event (HAE) is most commonly a Root Cause Analysis (RCA) to find factors and conditions that caused or contributed to the HAE. The basis for the RCA is the James Reason Swiss Cheese model of adverse events developed from analysis of large-scale industrial accidents. In this model the HAE occurs when a patient deteriorating clinical trajectory broaches the hospital's organisational and professional defences. The learnings from the RCA typically result in new or changed policies and procedures, and occasionally professional disciplinary review of the involved health care workers. Clinical Futile Cycles (CFC) is clinical action or intervention (or lack thereof) that has no patient benefit. Analysis of HAE by looking for CFC creates learnings that focus on the human factors of the involved health care workers, and more importantly the socio, politico, and fiscal cultural hospital environment at the time of the HAE. As such, the learnings focus not on limitations of the individual practitioners but rather, the greater environment that has them often ignoring, broaching or being oblivious to professional standards, and the already existent policy procedure and guidelines.

Keywords: Clinical Futile Cycles, hospital adverse events, Root Cause Analysis, hierarchical model of care

1. Introduction

When unexpected clinical deterioration results in patient harm (death or permanent disability), healthcare in an attempt to learn from its mistakes, uses Quality Improvement tools from other industries, principally Root Cause Analysis (RCA). RCA methodology takes a structured template of criteria that is applied objectively to the timeframe of the adverse event in question. The outcome of this process is a set of learnings for practice improvement. The purpose of this article is not to detract from

 IntechOpen

the process of RCA, rather to question why all too often despite, a RCA, the same mistakes are repeated often again and again. Indeed, overall, the incidence and outcomes from hospital adverse events (HAE), has not improved over the last two decades [1–6]. This is despite widespread recognition of the problem, extensive epidemiological research, and billions of dollars of investment into quality and safety programs [2, 3].

Clinical Futile Cycles is defined as clinical activity that has no nett benefit to the patient. Across all spheres of medical practice clinical activity is undertaken with no actual benefit to the patient but also that does no harm apart from cost. In the case of a patient's condition deteriorating clinical activity is needed to cure or at least improve the clinical situation. In the critically unstable patient, failure to improve the patient condition is equivalent to deterioration, due to the underlying principles of pathophysiology. Cellular homeostasis is dependent on adequate delivery of oxygen to mitochondria to sustain aerobic metabolism. Anaerobic metabolism due to blood loss, hypoxia, sepsis, cardiopulmonary pathology has to be reversed or the cell, and then an organ and eventually the body will die. As such it is imperative that in this type of clinical situation the clinical activity is productive in the restoration of homeostasis, not futile, to prevent the downward spiral to death or permanent disability.

In this article, the case for the examination of HAE, through a process of looking for and then examining the Clinical Futile Cycles that inevitably occur throughout patient deterioration is made [7, 8]. In doing so, the pandoras box of what really goes on at the interface between the deteriorating patient, the individual frontline health care workers, and finally and just as importantly, the socio, cultural, political nature of involved health care system and or hospital, is opened. Thus, the learnings are focused on changes that are needed to create productive clinical activity that improves patient outcomes. Finally using this model, some fundamental reforms for the prevention of these adverse events are proposed.

2. Limitations of RCA and the traditional "Swiss Cheese" model of healthcare and hospital setting adverse events

Attempts to reduce the incidence of adverse events and make hospitals safer have been largely unsuccessful [2, 4–6]. Like other diseases and conditions, an understanding of the underlying aetiology or "pathophysiology" of adverse events is important for the development of preventative strategies. To date the predominant theory to explain adverse events in health has been the "Swiss Cheese" model developed by James Reason from his analysis of large scale industrial and organisational accidents [9].

James Reason in his book "Managing the Risks of Organizational Accidents" states that organisational accidents, as opposed to individual accidents, are predictable events [9]. An individual accident is one in which a person or group of people makes an individual slip, lapse, or error of judgement with the net result being an adverse outcome either to the person or the people who erred, or to the person or people in the immediate vicinity. As such there is usually a relatively tight, simple explanation for cause and effect in an individual accident. On the other hand, organisational accidents have "multiple causes involving many people at different levels of an organization" [9]. These events, whilst usually infrequent, are often catastrophic. Analyses of such organisational accidents often reveal that the defences an organisation has to prevent such catastrophes are breached by a unique series of sequential hazards that play out in an environment of latent conditions, the so called "Swiss Cheese". It follows that, one can decrease the incidence of these organisational accidents by increasing the number of defences (more cheese slices) and/or by shrinking the size of the holes in each of the defences (**Figure 1**). This is the basis for the RCA investigation of a HAE.

In 2008, Palmieri et al. published their "Health Care Error Proliferation Model" of adverse healthcare events [10]. This model takes the "Swiss Cheese Model" and specifically adapts the various factors that exist in healthcare (**Figure 2**). Most notably, they place clinician vigilance as a key defence at the sharp end of the actual adverse event, in the form of clinical improvisation and localised workarounds. This clinician vigilance repairs gaps produced by actions, changes and adjustments that are made at the blunt end of the healthcare organisation with its administrative and therefore higher level, layers of defence. A good example of this is the use of high-definition mobile telephone devices in rural and regional settings that allow almost immediate transfer of clinical information to an appropriate clinician at a referral centre. However, this clinical workaround and improvisation is clearly at odds with most organisations' patient privacy policies that have been developed at the blunt administrative end of the organisation.

Having for the most part accepted the Reason "Swiss Cheese" model of adverse events and adapted variations, most hospitals response to adverse events has been to increase defences at the blunt end of the healthcare organisation's administration [3]. These defences, in the hospital, take the form of dedicated quality and safety units and committees, electronic event reporting systems, and the development of appropriate standards linked to hospital accreditation [3]. The aim of each of these blunt end defence layers is to continually decrease the size of the holes in each defence layer, by more audits, meetings, and RCA analysis projects combined with the use of the quality improvement cycle. Inevitably what is generated is recommendations, guidelines and more policy and procedure.

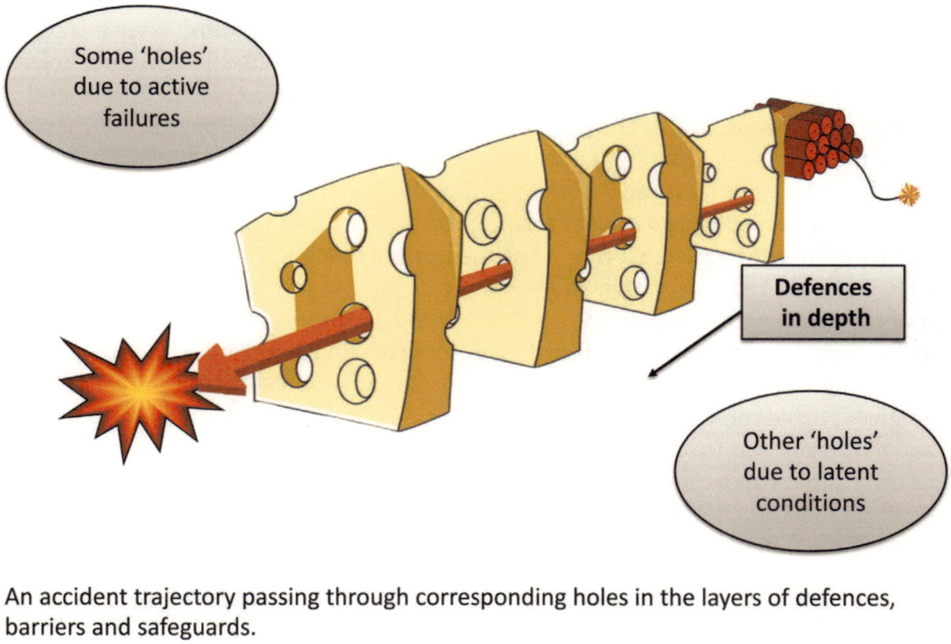

Figure 1.
The Reason "Swiss Cheese" model [22].

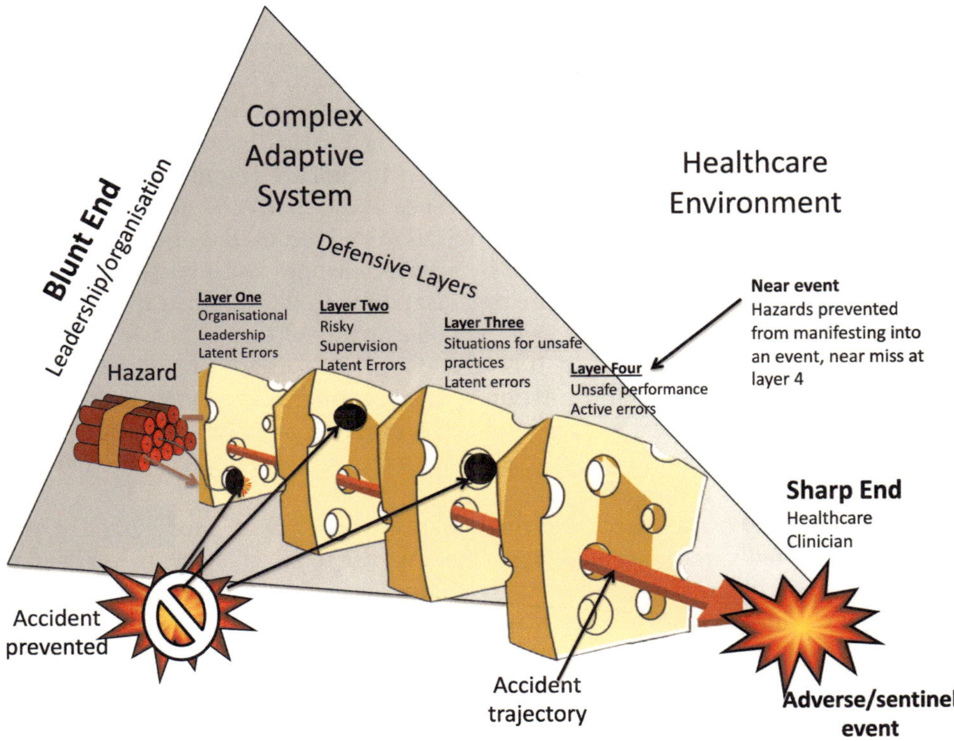

Figure 2.
Healthcare error proliferation model [25].

The "Swiss Cheese" model does explain well some types of hospital adverse events, in particular patient falls, wrong side surgery and medication errors. In the case of medication errors, root cause analysis of these events often highlights holes in the "Swiss Cheese," such as poor transcription of medication prescriptions, and failure to do appropriate checks [11]. In the case of patient falls, there is failure to identify the "at risk" patient and put in place appropriate preventative strategies. Fixing the holes or at least reducing the size of them can reduce the incidence of patient falls and medication errors. This can be done by and large with top-down policy and procedure and ensuring implementation of such [12]. The best example of this has been the reduction in incidence of wrong side surgery, with the implementation of time out, with completion of a check list before surgery [13]. The Reason "Swiss Cheese" model gives good explanation of the adverse event when there is a relatively tight temporal relationship, between the adverse event and preventative strategies. The adverse event itself in these circumstances is itself evidence that a mistake or error was made. There is usually with the "Swiss Cheese" model a series of clear errors that can be identified. This model then allows for preventative strategies to be implemented, and with the increasing move back to professional responsibility for compliance, in theory at least the Holy Grail of the perfectly safe hospital should be attainable.

However, most adverse events in hospital, particularly the more serious ones, often do not have such clear errors with a tight temporal relationship with the adverse event and the contributing errors. When the temporal relationship between the adverse event and the preventative strategies is not so tight, hospital cultural factors start to be more significant, and the potential for policy and procedure to help is much less so, simply because it can be and often is ignored.

3. Problems with RCA and the "Swiss Cheese" model: why are hospitals different from other industries?

There are three fundamental problems with the application of the "Swiss Cheese" model to adverse events in hospitals. First, in the hospital, the distinction between individual and organisational accidents is not clear. The entire premise of the "Swiss Cheese" model was the investigation of causation factors of large industrial accidents as opposed to individual accidents. In the hospital we do not have large scale accidents but, instead, multiple little accidents or adverse events daily, if not hourly, and in almost every setting. The literature on causation of adverse events in hospitals overwhelmingly points to failures at the sharp end of care delivery to the patient by frontline staff. Analysis of the causative factors associated with the adverse events in The Quality in Australian Health Care Study found that cognitive failure was a factor in 57% of these adverse events [14]. In this analysis, cognitive failure included such errors as: failure to synthesise, decide and act on available information; failure to request or arrange an investigation, procedure or consultation; lack of care or attention; failure to attend; misapplication of, or failure to apply, a rule, or use of a bad or inadequate rule [14]. In a two-hospital study from the United Kingdom that looked at 100 sequential admissions to the intensive care unit (ICU) from ward areas, it was found that 54 had sub-optimal care on the ward prior to transfer [15]. This group of patients had a mortality rate of 56%. Some of the sub-optimal treatment factors included failure to seek advice, lack of knowledge, failure to appreciate clinical urgency, and lack of supervision [15].

Adoption of the Reason "Swiss Cheese" model for organisational accidents has led the whole Quality and Safety industry, and in particular hospitals, looking for system solutions to what can be explained by individual competency and micro environment cultural issues at the patient interface. In particular, a major rationale of Reason's philosophy is to avoid individual accountability for errors and the culture of blame and shame. Nearly 20 years ago Reason himself noted the folly of this approach in medicine when he stated, "*It is curious that such a bastion of discretionary action as medicine should be moving towards a 'Feed Forward' mode of control when many other hitherto rule dominated domains – notably railways and oil exploration and production – are shifting towards performance-based controls and away from prescriptive ones*" [9]. When Reason talks about human contribution to organisational accidents, he describes two schemas of control [9]. A "Feed Forward" control system is one where human performance is determined by rules and procedures as determined by an organisational standards and objectives. In this schema occasional accidents and incidents are analysed and then fed back into either an alteration of an existing rule or procedure or the creation of a new one (**Figure 3**). At the other end of the control spectrum there is the model where organisational output is largely determined by individual human performance. The basis for this model is that, in the first instance, the humans are generally highly trained and that performance is controlled by continual performance reinforcement against a known or standard comparator (**Figure 4**). The best example of this, in hospitals, is specialist medical practice. To even start specialist training there have been many years of training and experience (medical school, house officer jobs, and pre specialty registrar placements) followed by a period of mentoring

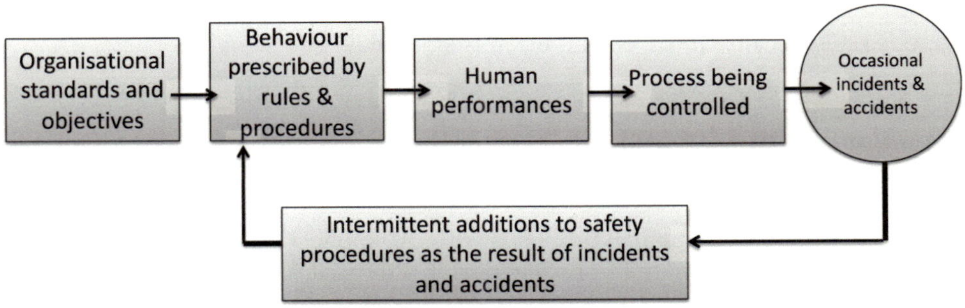

Figure 3.
The Reason Feedforward process control system [22].

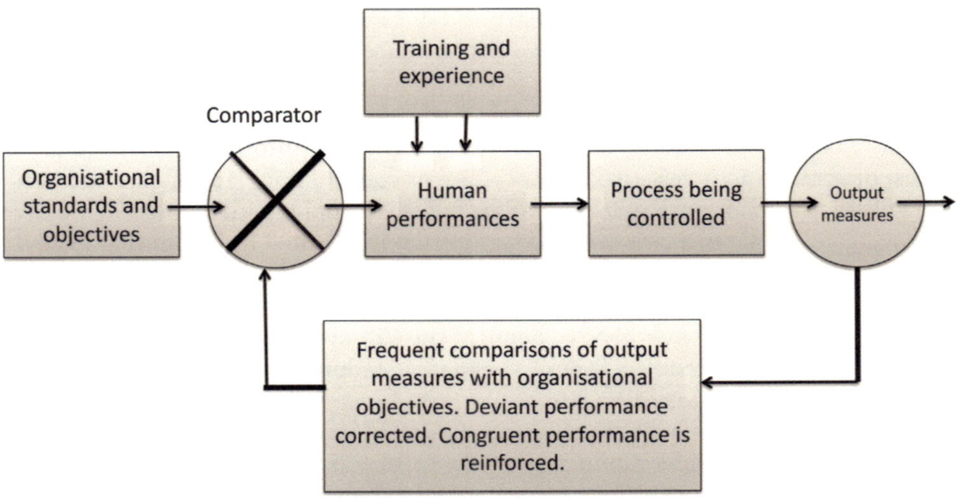

Figure 4.
The Reason feedback process control system [22].

and in essence apprenticeship to learn the specialty to the known standard of the comparator, the standard of practice as maintained by the specialty colleges. Taking these two schemata one can immediately see the trouble with health care in hospitals. It is a large industry with community and political expectations that are more congruent with the "Feed Forward" schema, but yet with most of the actual clinical activity being undertaken by the "Human Performance" schema.

What we have seen in the construction of hospital adverse event defences is an over reliance on the administrative blunt end of the organisation, in terms of policy and procedures, with the assumption that the health care professionals at the patient end are competent and will be compliant. The shift to looking for hospital wide problems has come at the cost of avoiding the issue of individual professional accountability and associated issues, most notably the education and certification of health care professionals. In Australia and the United Kingdom, several studies indicate that the medical undergraduate syllabus does not provide graduates with the basic knowledge, skills, and judgement to manage acute life-threatening emergencies [16–18]. These studies identified deficiencies in cognitive abilities, procedural skills, and communication. Despite this, undergraduate and postgraduate curricula have been slow to embrace a patient safety culture [19–21].

The second fundamental problem with the "Swiss Cheese" model and the Palmieri variation of this are, that they are overly simplistic and do not take into account the complexity of the patient and the hospital system. When a patient enters a hospital system, they enter a system where they will be exposed to a variety of hazards which, in turn, have numerous defences in place to prevent an adverse patient outcome. Operations, anaesthesia, medical interventions and procedures, drugs and fluids and even oxygen therapy constitute the hazards. Most defences in health care are reliant on the competence of the health care professional and as such are "soft." "Hard" defences are those that are impossible to overcome, for example in anaesthesia where the administration of hypoxic gas mixtures is physically prevented. The soft defences, in health care include treatment policies and procedures, manual alarm systems, and ad hoc hierarchical and lateral human checking systems. Soft defences are very reliant on the training and education that healthcare workers receive and the culture of compliance. Superimposed on these layers of hazards and defences that confront a patient, there are the latent conditions that exist, most obviously within the patient, but more insidiously within the hospital as an organisation. A patient's past medical history, family history, social history, associated co-morbidities, drug regimen and allergies largely constitute their latent conditions. These conditions and their relation to the current presenting complaint that brings the patient into the hospital system, is territory that individual healthcare workers are usually extremely well trained in and familiar with. Hospital latent conditions are not so explicit, particularly to the patient or the frontline healthcare worker. They are made up of a complex matrix of production and cultural imperatives such as the financial operating environment, political and societal imperatives, medico-legal and insurance concerns, compliance issues imposed by various regulatory bodies (often with associated financial incentives or disincentives) and workforce and work-practice issues. Thus, in the hospital system, unlike any other industry we have a high degree of ever-changing complexity; complex patients and a complex system where adverse events are essentially prevented by a whole host of predominantly soft defences [22]. The "Swiss Cheese" model is a static model with fixed defences in terms of the layers and the size of holes in each layer. This translates well into most industries, but in health care, the complexity is dynamic and ever changing, the number of holes and layers change with every patient and each and every different healthcare professional.

The third problem with the "Swiss Cheese" model is that adverse events in hospitals occur so insidiously that they become normalised into the operating behaviour and practice of the organisation. This is distinct from large scale industrial accidents, where the impact of the event has a high degree of face validity, primarily due to the immediacy and scale of the event. Therefore, in terms of numbers, patient adverse events may constitute a crisis. However, to the individual practitioner or even hospital these events may not appear to be a problem. On the whole, such events are infrequent and occur, over a long-time frame. For example, The Quality in Australian Healthcare Study looked at a random sample of 14,179 admissions to 28 hospitals in two states of Australia in 1992 and documented 112 deaths (0.79%) and 109 cases where the adverse event caused greater than 50% disability (0.77%) [14]. Seventy percent of the deaths and 58% of the cases of significant disability were considered to have had a high degree of preventability [14]. Thus, for the individual clinicians, treating departments and units, and even the 28 study hospitals themselves, their actual experience of these outcomes, over the year would be minimal (one or two cases) [14].

The "Swiss Cheese" model and RCA gives a poor explanation of the multitude of insidious individual accidents that occur in hospitals and is too simplistic for the complexity of most patients and the complex matrix of healthcare that is provided in a hospital. Most importantly, the focus on system issues whilst valid and important, has detracted from what is really needed; focussed attention on clinical competence and accountability at the patient interface.

4. Clinical Futile Cycles and the traditional hierarchical referral model of care

The term "Futile Cycle" is a term used in cell biology and biochemistry to explain the conversion of one substance to another and back to the original substance by two always on enzymatic pathways. However, despite the enzymatic activity and energy utilisation there is no net output or gain from this energy consuming and active process. This is exactly what we see with hospital patient adverse events, and in particular the deteriorating patient; a lot of clinical activity, none of which effectively alters the trajectory of the patient in the downward spiral to the HAE. The clinical activity occurs in a traditional hierarchal referral model of care that by its very nature is often either unresponsive or slowly responsive and where the exhaustive policy and procedures are often ignored.

In the hospital, the "Clinical Futile Cycle" usually starts with the most junior level of the "traditional hierarchical referral model of care," at the bedside with the interaction between the junior nurse and the patient (**Figure 5**). With a clinical abnormality, be it an observation, a wrong drug order, or a procedural failure, the junior nurse must make a decision as to the significance of the abnormality and the importance of

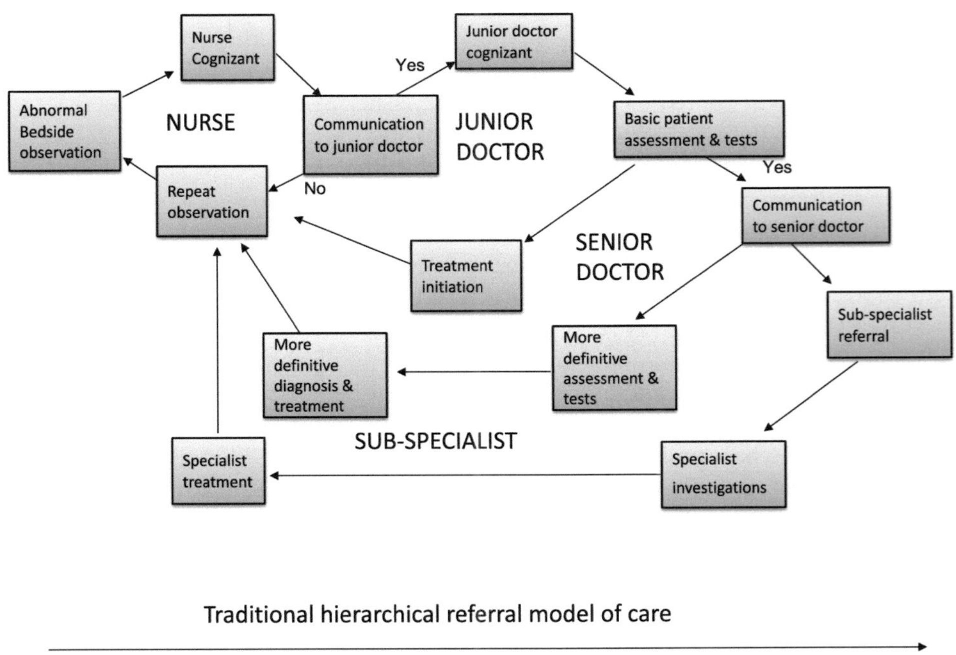

Figure 5.
Clinical Futile Cycles [23, 24].

reporting it to a more senior team member, either a senior nurse or the most available (usually junior) doctor. However, that decision to escalate the issue can be influenced the workplace culture that exists in the particular micro environment of that bedside and that ward at that time [23]. If the concern or abnormality is escalated, it is to the next person in the care hierarchy of the team looking after that patient. This is often the junior doctor who then needs to attend, assess and then also make a decision about whether or not to escalate the issue to the next person in the hierarchy. This is important because, for the most, the junior doctor does not have the skills or emotional intelligence to appropriately manage a lot of these clinical abnormalities [32–35]. If the issue is escalated, it is often to a middle grade doctor, one who is often a specialist in training and who as such may be difficult to find. Unlike their juniors, usually this grade of doctor does have the technical and clinical abilities to deal with the particular issue. However, they are often over committed with clinics, operating theatre, and ward rounds. Additionally, this grade of doctor is diagnosis focused and often we see them giving instructions to their juniors (usually appropriately) to organise specialised investigations and other speciality consultations. There is nothing wrong with this, except for the fact that it is time consuming (**Figure 6**) [24].

In support of the "Clinical Futile Cycles" model is the literature that has looked at the causation of adverse events in hospitals [14, 15, 25, 26]. All these studies can assign almost all causation to three human factor issues at the patient interface; competency, cognition (or failure thereof) and culture. Perhaps the most disturbing example of this was described in the MERIT study; a randomised cluster control study of Medical Emergency Teams (MET) [27] in 23 Australian hospitals (including private and rural hospitals) in 2002. In the nearly 500 cardiac arrests that occurred during the study, in more than a third of instances staff took abnormal (that broached MET activation criteria) patient observations in the 15 min prior to the cardiac arrest, but did not activate an emergency response. The first thing of note with this phenomenon was that the incidence of not calling for help in an abnormal patient situation was high at 30% in the intervention hospitals, and 40% in the control hospitals. Put another way,

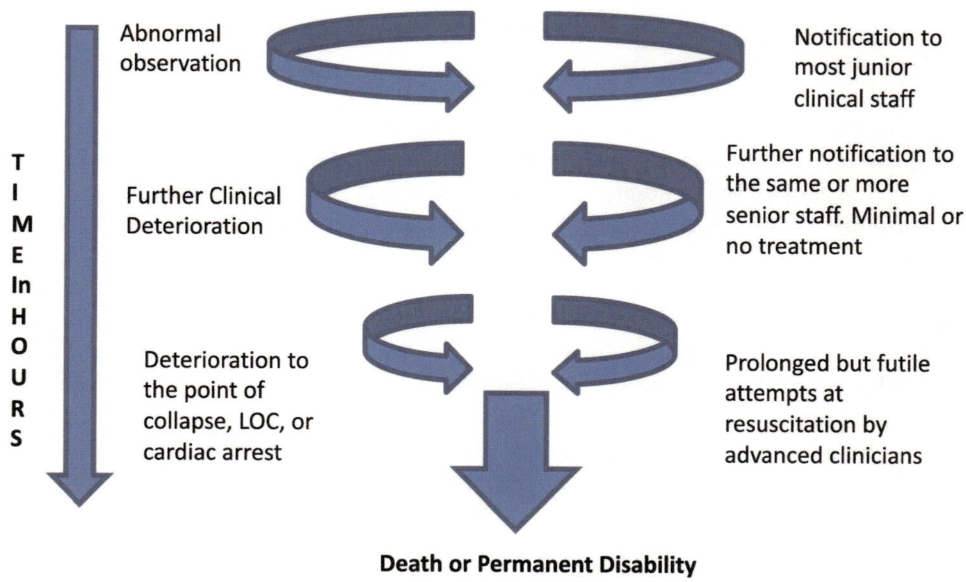

Figure 6.
The downward spiral of Clinical Futile Cycles in the deteriorating patient.

in the average Australian hospital in 2002, if a patient had documented abnormal signs, in the 15 min before a cardiac arrest, in up to 40% of the time the staff did nothing about this. Another thing of note with these findings is that in intervention hospitals that had had an intense education process on the new MET activation policy and procedure, the incidence of calling for help was only 10% greater than the control hospitals [27]. It is here at the bedside with the pre cardiac arrest patient that the staff are trapped in a clinical futile cycle, unable to get out of it due to either clinical incompetency (not able to recognise and act for the pre arrest patient) and/or culture whereby calling for help maybe considered not the norm in that ward, on that shift at that time [28–30].

The "Swiss Cheese" response when RRS fail at the sharp end, or afferent limb failure (ALF), the response is to assume policy and procedure failure, with hospital administrations, all too often, is just to alter the policy and procedure and make the activation criteria mandatory for the bedside staff [31]. This is done without areal understanding of what actually is going on at the bedside, the various heath care worker interactions and the overall socio-cultural environment of the hospital. Despite the intuitive appeal of Rapid Response Systems [32] their potential benefits [33] have been limited by this phenomenon of ALF [34]. In essence the RRS resuscitation teams cannot benefit the deteriorating patient if they are not notified about them. The incidence of bedside staff failure to activate the RRS has been measured at between 17 and 68% albeit that the various studies have used different criteria, definitions and methodologies [29, 34, 35]. What may be going on is that here may be problem with the face validity of RRS due to the very low specificity of the activation criteria [36–38]. Furthermore, there may be problems around staff competency, or cultural issues around staff losing face by calling for help. As a result, rather than trying to understand or deal with this very real issue of face validity, possible competency issues and probable cultural issues, the administrative response, is usually simplistic.

5. Using Clinical Futile Cycles to safety proof health from the sharp end back

If we accept the model of clinical futile cycles, it becomes immediately apparent that no amount of activity away from the sharp end of the healthcare adverse event will help, least of all the generation of more policy and procedure. Instead, we need to focus attention on the healthcare professional and the immediate socio-cultural environment in which they work [39]. Dealing first with the health care worker; the selection of these individuals to undertake their chosen vocation is invariably done by consideration of various personal attributes, in the case of medicine academic achievement and individual performance in tests [40–43]. This process and subsequent education take no account of the fact that as soon as these people graduate, they will be working in a team environment.

The clinical care we deliver (and receive) is a function of the education and capability of our students who will eventually be our doctors and ultimately clinical leaders and decision makers. What we teach and practise best is point of care medicine and clinical interventions. Therefore, it is no surprise that what we examine and, and what students focus on, is specific point of care clinical assessments and interventions [44]. This is best represented by the objective, structured, clinical, examination system (OSCE) that is now a widespread and common form of summative assessment

[45]. In the OSCE, candidates undertake clinical assessment tasks at a number of specific stations for 5–8 min. Each station has a structured "score card" that students must address to get the points. This system of examination in no way gives any indication on a student's ability and competency to comprehensively take a history, do a physical examination, synthesise these findings into a meaningful problem list and finally and actually least importantly come up with a diagnosis [46]. It has got to the point now in the undergraduate curriculum, that the clinical process of whole patient assessment is variably taught and certainly not examined, in a sufficiently stringent manner to motivate students to spend long hours doing patient histories and examinations. Having competent health care professionals spend time with and understanding our patients is the single biggest step to making health care safe.

Second, priority needs to be given to the core business of hospital care; the interaction at the bedside and clinic between the patient and the various healthcare professionals [28–30]. Clinical Futile Cycles gives a practical platform to understand this culture. We need to accept that an abnormal or inappropriate workplace culture is at the heart of every major inquiry into poor hospital care [47–52]. Every report into these enquiries recommends change. Yet 30 years on from Bristol [51] we have mid-Staffordshire [50]. So, what have we really learned from the reports and thousands of pages of recommendations? Nothing. We need a different strategy; one that puts the patient and their wellbeing first. This should be followed by the implicit understanding that our core business is that of interaction with the patient from the most basic and junior levels. The bedside healthcare team needs to be trained, credentialed and supported to deliver better healthcare, not as individual players, but as members of a team (**Table 1**).

	RCA	CFC
Scope	Limited to timeline of patient episode of care	As for RCA, but examines workplace culture, interaction between healthcare staff, in the hierarchical hospital system and takes account of socio, cultural, fiscal and political factors
Causation	Broken into categories of, Communication, Task, Equipment, Patient and Care team and organisation	As above plus, human factors, education, and administration
Recommendations	Attempts to fill in the holes in the "Swiss Cheese" model of causation	Assumes that either the holes in the "Swiss Cheese" will reoccur or that new ones will be made. Aims to address issues of competence with individual practitioners, culture of practice between practitioners, and the influence of the organisations fiscal political and social environment
Outcomes	Changes to Policy and Procedure Professional disciplinary action against the bedside practitioners	Addresses limitations in Human Factors at an individual practitioner level Monitors addresses abnormal cultural practices at a ward and department level Assumption of responsibility for socio, politico, fiscal factors by organisation administration and government

Table 1.
Hospital adverse events; review by root cause analysis (RCA) versus clinical futile cycles (CFC).

5.1 Two typical cases

References

https://www.abc.net.au/news/2021-05-17/aishwarya-aswath-perth-childrens-hospital-death-report-released/100144052 (last viewed 22/07/2021)

On April the 3rd 2021 at 1722 a 7-year-old child girl presented to the Emergency Department at Perth Children's Hospital (PCH). Prior to death the family made multiple attempts to get help, which did not occur, despite continuing and deteriorating signs of sepsis. At 2122 after more than an hour of resuscitation she was deceased. The following morning a blood culture grew Strep A. In the ensuing days weeks and months, several of the frontline clinical staff have been referred to APHRA, in retaliation the Nurses union have referred several middle level nurse managers to APHRA. The Chairperson of the PCH resigned, the CEO offered his resignation, and there have been calls for the State Health minister to resign. An initial confidential RCA report into the death highlighted many short comings and made 11 recommendations that were tabled in Parliament. The family rejected the findings as contradictory. They have insisted that such a death should never occur again. Reportedly morale amongst staff at the hospital and in particular the Emergency department is at a "rock bottom low."

WA's Child and Adolescent Health Service (CAHS) will not endorse its own report into a 7-year-old's death at Perth Children's Hospital until an independent investigation has been completed.

Key points

- Health executives say further investigations are needed
- The 7-year-old died after waiting for treatment at PCH
- An independent review into her death is being prepared

The report, which was released by Aishwarya Aswath's family, detailed what happened the night Aishwarya died, including the response from staff, as she waited around 2 h to be treated before being declared dead just after 9:00 pm on Saturday, April 3.

The CAHS review was conducted by a panel that was made up of a mix of health department employees and external experts.

"The panel found there were a cascade of missed opportunities to address parental concerns and incomplete assessments, with a delay in escalation which may have contributed to the patient's outcome," the report found.

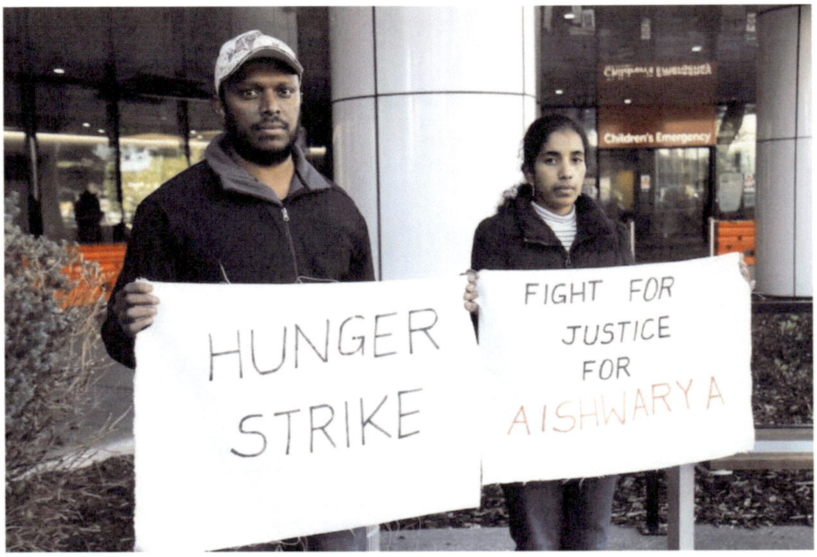

Aishwarya's parents Aswath Chavittupara and Prasitha Sasidharan released the report to the public.*(ABC News: West Matteeussen).*

Eleven recommendations were made, including improvement to the triage process policy at PCH, a clear pathway for parents to escalate concerns to staff, a review of cultural awareness for staff and development of an established sepsis recognition diagnostic tool in the emergency department.

The state government has promised there will also be an independent inquiry into the hospital's emergency department, and a coronial inquest into Aishwarya's death.

More investigations needed: CAHS

CAHS chief executive Aresh Anwar said he agreed with Aishwarya's family that she was not shown compassion and care.

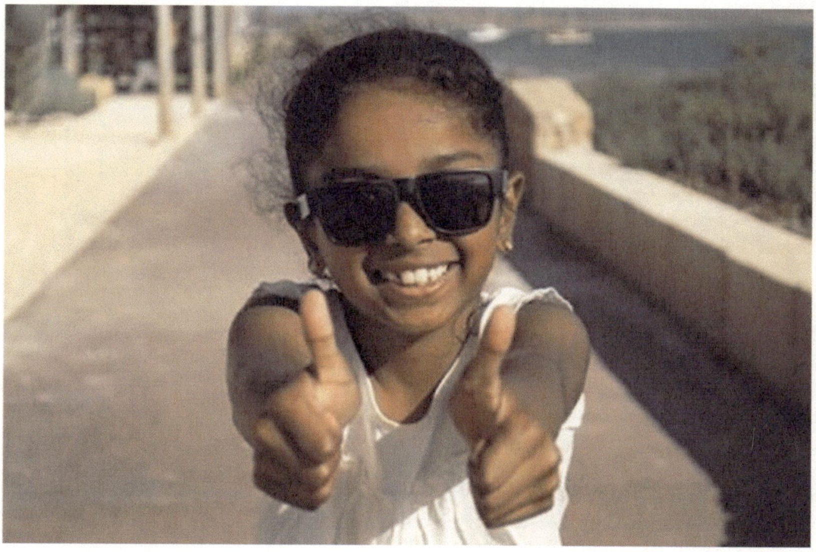

Aishwarya Aswath died after waiting for treatment at Perth Children's Hospital's emergency department. *(Supplied: Family).*

But he said the report would not be endorsed until further investigations were completed.

"The CAHS Executive acknowledge the findings of the panel," Dr. Anwar said in a statement provided to the ABC.

"The report represents a significant volume of investigation," however, it is the opinion of the CAHS executive that there are a number of elements that require further exploration.

"The additional independent external review must be completed before we can, in good conscience," consider this investigation to be finalised.

"This additional targeted review will ensure" we fully understand the opportunities for systemic change.

"While we await the additional independent external review," we are not in a position to endorse this root cause analysis report.

"However, we remain committed and are urgently implementing all 11 recommendations."

Health Minister Roger Cook warned against making conclusions about the circumstances surrounding Aishwarya's death before additional investigations were carried out.

"We need to make sure that as individuals we don't try to play judge and jury in relation to what happened in the ED on the night Aishwarya passed away," he said.

"We weren't there, we don't know, so it's important that we leave it up to the experts and make sure they get the opportunity to investigate this properly."

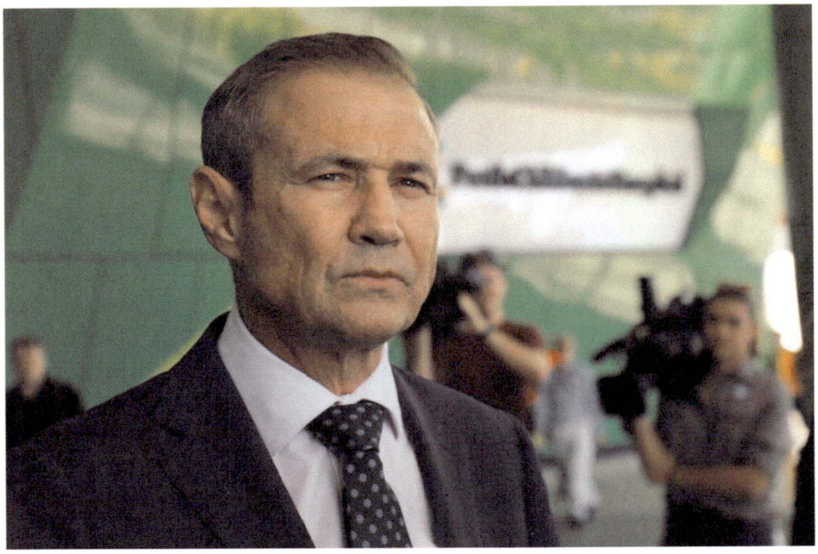

Health Minister Roger Cook says he wants to ensure nurses feel "heard and supported". *(ABC News: Eliza Laschon).*

The Minister met with doctors and nurses at PCH's emergency department this afternoon.

"This will be my opportunity to tell them that I support them in the difficult work they do," he said.

"I want them to know that we will continue to work hard to make sure they have the resources they need to do the job that they are committed to."

"I'm committed to work with them closely, to come back as often as they feel necessary to make sure they feel heard and supported."

Staff 'upset' with Minister at meeting

The meeting was also attended by the Australian Nursing Federation WA chief executive Mark Olson and Australian Medical Association WA president Andrew Miller.

Emerging from the meeting, Dr. Miller said it had become emotional, with staff taking the opportunity to "call it how it is" in front of the Health Minister.

"He was received, I would say, poorly," he said.

"I've never heard staff quite so upset with anyone in a meeting before that they would speak out in that way."

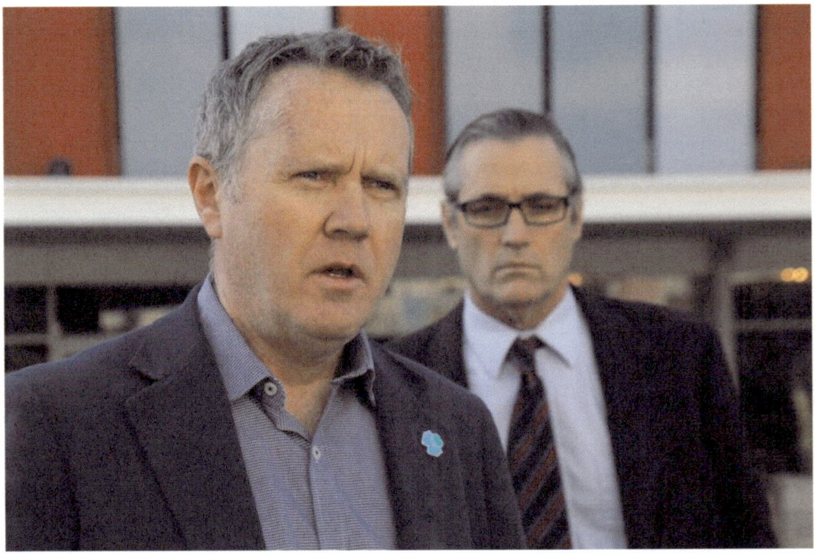

AMA WA president Andrew Miller (left) says staff took the opportunity to "call it how it is". *(ABC News: Eliza Laschon).*

Dr. Miller said staff were particularly upset by reports some of their colleagues would be referred to the medical regulator, the Australian Health Practitioner Regulation Agency (AHPRA).

In response, he said he intended to make his own referrals to the watchdog.

"It's pretty clear from the evasion that we heard from management that they are intending [to], or have, reported very junior members of the staff to AHPRA," Dr. Miller said.

"We have expressed our dismay and disgust over that."

"If that if that proceeds, [I intend to] report the registered managers, executives and the director-general involved in setting up the system within which these junior staff work, so that AHPRA has the opportunity to consider everyone's actions in this."

Mr. Olson said during the meeting, nurses again raised concerns about staffing levels in the emergency department, both on the night Aishwarya died and since.

"There is this disconnect between those who are running the hospital and those who are working in the hospital," he said.

"[The nurses] have no faith in the executive at the moment. They have no trust that the executive can rebuild the reputation and rebuild the trust that the community needs in this hospital, and it's taking a toll."

Posted 20 May 2021 20 May 2021, updated 20 May 2021 20 May 2021.

Box 1.
Death of Aishwarya Aswath at Perth Children's Hospital, Australia, April 2021.

References

https://www.pulsetoday.co.uk/analysis/regulation/bawa-garba-timeline-of-a-case-that-has-rocked-medicine/ (last viewed 28/07/2021)

18 February 2011

A 6 year old boy is admitted to the Children's Assessment Unit (CAU) at Leicester Royal Infirmary following a referral from his GP. Jack Adcock, who had Down's Syndrome and a known heart condition, had been suffering from diarrhoea, vomiting and had difficulty breathing.

Dr. Hadiza Bawa-Garba was a specialist registrar in year six of her postgraduate training (ST6) with an 'impeccable' record. She had recently returned from maternity leave and this was her first shift in an acute setting. She was the most senior doctor covering the CAU, the emergency department and the ward CAU that day. She saw Jack at about 10.30 am.

Jack was receiving supplementary oxygen and Dr. Bawa-Garba prescribed a fluid bolus and arranged for blood tests and a chest x-ray. At 10.44 am the first blood gas test was available and showed a worryingly high lactate reading. The x-ray became available from around 12.30 pm and showed evidence of a chest infection.

Dr. Bawa-Garba was heavily involved in treating other children between 12 and 3 pm, including a baby that needed a lumbar puncture. At 3 pm Dr. Bawa-Garba reviewed Jack's X-ray (she was not informed before then that it was available) and prescribed a dose of antibiotics immediately, which Jack received an hour later from the nurses.

A failure in the hospital's electronic computer system that day meant that although she had ordered blood tests at about 10.45 am, Dr. Bawa-Garba did not receive them until about 4.15 pm. It also meant her senior house office was unavailable.

During a handover meeting with a consultant which took place about 4.30 pm, Dr. Bawa-Garba raised the high level of CRP in Jack's blood test results and a diagnosis of pneumonia, but she did not ask the consultant to review the patient. She said Jack had been much improved and was bouncing about. At 6.30 pm, she spoke to the consultant a second time, but again did not raise any concerns.

When she wrote up the initial notes, she did not specify that Jack's enalapril (for his heart condition) should be discontinued. Jack was subsequently given his evening dose of enalapril by his mother after he was transferred to the ward around 7 pm.

At 8 pm a 'crash call' went out and Dr. Bawa-Garba was one of the doctors who responded to it. On entering the room she mistakenly confused Jack with another patient and called off the resuscitation. Her mistake was identified within 30 s to 2 min and resuscitation continued.

This hiatus did not contribute to Jack's death, as his condition was already too far advanced. At 9.20 pm, Jack died.

2 November 2015

Portuguese agency nurse, 47-year-old Isabel Amaro, of Manchester is given a 2-year suspended gaol sentence for manslaughter on the grounds of gross negligence.

4 November 2015

At Nottingham Crown Court Dr. Bawa-Garba is convicted of manslaughter on the grounds of gross negligence.

14 December 2015

Dr. Bawa-Garba is given a 24 month suspended sentence.

8 December 2016

Dr. Bawa-Garba's appeal against her sentence is quashed at the Court of Appeal.

13 June 2017

The Medical Practitioners Tribunal service says Dr. Bawa-Garba should be suspended for 12 months and rejects an application from the GMC to strike her off the register. It says: 'In the circumstances of this case, balancing the mitigating and aggravating factors, the tribunal concluded that erasure would be disproportionate.'

8 December 2017

GMC takes the MPTS to the High Court and argues its own tribunal was 'wrong' to allow Dr Bawa-Garba to continue to practise.

25 January 2018

The GMC successfully appeals at the High Court bid to have the MPTS decision overruled, leading to Dr. Bawa-Garba being struck off the medical register. Lord Justice Ouseley says: 'The Tribunal did not respect the verdict of the jury as it should have. In fact, it reached its own and less severe view of the degree of Dr Bawa-Garba's personal culpability.' Health secretary Jeremy Hunt says that he is 'deeply concerned' about its implications.

26 January 2018

Prominent GPs tell Pulse that the ruling raises serious questions about how doctor's reflections are used and recorded, and that new guidance is now needed urgently.

30 January 2018

An influential international doctors group accuses the GMC of treating black and minority ethnic doctors 'differently and harshly', following the High Court case.

In light of the Dr. Bawa-Garba case, the GMC announces a review of how gross negligence manslaughter is applied to medical practice, which was initially led by Dame Clare Marx and later taken over by Leslie Hamilton after Dame Clare was appointed the next GMC chair. Meanwhile, an influential international doctors group accuses the GMC of treating black and minority ethnic doctors 'differently and harshly', following the High Court case.

31 January 2018

Dr. Bawa-Garba's defence body releases a statement saying e-portfolio reflections were not used against her in court, despite 'wide misreporting' that they were. But Pulse uncovers that her reflections were used in court, from a document submitted as evidence by the on-call consultant on the day.

6 February 2018

Former health secretary Jeremy Hunt announces a review into the application of gross negligence manslaughter charges in medicine in light of the Dr Bawa-Garba case.

7 February 2018

Following a crowd funding campaign, which raised over £335,000, Dr. Bawa-Garba decides to appeal the ruling, and considers appealing the manslaughter conviction from 2015.

12 February 2018

The GMC refutes claims that there was discrimination in its decision to launch a High Court bid. In response to an open letter from the British Association of Physicians of Indian Origin (BAPIO), the GMC said the accusations were 'troubling and without merit'.

19 February 2018

The GMC is criticised by their regulator, the Professional Standards Authority (PSA), for striking off Dr. Bawa-Garba from the medical register. The PSA said the bid was 'without merit', according to an unpublished review of the case.

13 March 2018

GMC chair Professor Terence Stephenson says he is 'extremely sorry'for the distress caused to the medical profession by the Dr. Bawa-Garba case.

19 March 2018

University Hospitals of Leicester NHS Trust releases its serious incident report in to the death of Jack Adcock, which was completed 6 months after his death. The report says that there was no 'single root cause' behind the 6-year-old's death.

29 March 2018

Dr. Bawa-Garba is granted permission to appeal the High Court's decision to allow the GMC to strike of the junior doctor. Meanwhile, the BMA applies and is later permitted to advise the Court of Appeal in the case.

23 April 2018

The GMC announces the launch of its review into why black and minority ethnic doctors are more likely to face complaints from employers than their white colleagues, which is to be co-led by researcher Roger Kline and Dr. Doyin Atewologun.

11 June 2018

Department of Health and Social Care's 'rapid review' into medical gross negligence manslaughter concludes that the GMC should longer be able to appeal decisions made by its own tribunal regarding fitness-to-practise decisions.

27 June 2018

The BMA supports a vote of no confidence in the GMC in light of the Bawa-Garba case at its Annual Representative Meeting.

3 July 2018

Despite the conclusions of the DHSC's 'rapid review' in gross negligence manslaughter, the GMC tells Pulse it is not intending to halt appeals against its own fitness-to-practise tribunal until the law is changed.

25–26 July 2018

Dr. Bawa-Garba's appeal of the High Court decision that saw her struck off the medical register is heard in the High Court over one and a half days. Dr. Bawa-Garba said after the hearing that she is 'whole-heartedly sorry' for her mistakes, while Jack's mother Nicola Adcock says she 'will cause a public uproar' if Dr Bawa-Garba is reinstated.

13 August 2018

The Court of Appeal judges rule in favour of Dr Bawa-Garba, restoring the MPTS decision that she should be suspended from the medical register rather than erased. The judges said the matter has been passed to the MPTS 'for review of Dr Bawa-Garba's suspension'.

20 December 2018

The Medical Practitioner Tribunal Service (MPTS) decides to extend the suspension of Dr. Hadiza Bawa-Garba by a further 6 months, saying the measure is 'appropriate' to 'protect the public'.

13 March 2019

The MPTS announces a two-day review hearing for Dr. Bawa-Garba set for 8 and 9 April 2019. The hearing will decide whether her fitness to practise remains impaired and whether she is deemed fit to return to work.

8 April 2019

The MPTS rules that Dr. Bawa-Garba' the fitness to practise remains impaired, due to her lack of face-to-face patient contact while she was under suspension, agreeing that the risk of her putting another patient at an unwarranted risk of harm is low.

9 April 2019

The MPTS decides that Dr. Bawa-Garba will be able to return to practice from July 2019—under certain conditions—but she does not intend to return to work until February 2020, when her maternity leave finishes. The MPTS argues that the public interest has been served already by her cumulative suspension and that any higher sanction would be 'disproportionate and punitive'.

Sources

Mr Justice Nicol, Court of Appeal (Criminal Division), 8 December 2016

Medical Practitioner Tribunal Service Decision Dr Bawa-Garba. MPTS. 13 June 2017

High Court, December 2017—Reports from court reporter

MPTS press releases, 8–9 April 2019

For more on the Bawa-Garba case—click here

Box 2.
Death of Jack Adcock at Leicester Royal Infirmary, UK, February 2011.

6. Conclusion

After over three decades of the Quality and Safety movement two major themes are apparent. First, despite the best of efforts at an individual patient level, ward or department, hospital and organisation, the incidence of HAE has not substantively diminished. Second, the same mistakes are repeated. The traditional response to HAE has been the RCA and thence implementation of recommendations. This approach takes no or minimal account of the human factors involved or the socio, politico, fiscal and cultural circumstance that might be at play. At best this approach makes the assumption that such implementation will actually occur. At worst individual practitioners, usually junior, usually at the bedside, must take the responsibility and with it an unwieldy professional disciplinary process. There is rarely professional accountability for those further up the traditional hospital hierarchy despite their obvious engagement in setting the socio, political and fiscal arrangements for the organisation. Of greater concern they are often oblivious to particular sub optimal cultural practices that are often present when HAE's occur.

Clinical Futile Cycles gives an alternative framework to examine HAE, by directing focus at the futile clinical activity, and then trying to understand why such futile clinical activity occurred. With this understanding, interventions that target the early recognition of futile activity with the ultimate aim of learning clinical processes that are productive in circumventing clinical deterioration.

Author details

Michael Buist[1*] and Georgia Arnold[2]

1 College of Health and Medicine, University of Tasmania, Australia

2 Rural Clinical School, University of Tasmania, Australia

*Address all correspondence to: michael.buist@utas.edu.au

References

[1] Lunevicius R, Haagsma J. Incidence and mortality from adverse effects of medical treatment in the UK, 1990–2013: Levels, trends, patterns and comparision. International Journal for Quality in Health Care. 2018;**30**(7):558-564

[2] Shojania KG, Thomas EJ. Trends in adverse events over time: Why are we not improving. BMJ Quality and Safety. 2013;**22**:273-277. DOI: 10.1136/bmjqs-2013-001935

[3] Buist M, Middleton S. What went wrong with the quality and safety agenda? An essay by Michael Buist and Sarah Middleton. BMJ. 2013;**347**:f5800

[4] Landridge CP, Parry GJ, Bones CB, Hackbarth AD, Goldman DA, Sharek PJ. Temporal trends in rates of patient harm resulting from medical care. The New England Journal of Medicine. 2010;**363**: 2124-2134

[5] Classen DC, Resar R, Griffin F, Frederico F, Frankel T, Kimmel N, et al. Global trigger tool shows that adverse events in hospitals may be ten times greater than previously measured. Health AFF (Millwood). 2011;**30**:581-589

[6] Baines RJ, Langelaan M, de Bruijne MC, Spreeuwenberg P, Wagner C. Changes in adverse events in hospitals overtime: A longitudinal retrospective patient record review study. BMJ Quality and Safety. 2013;**22**:290-298

[7] Buist M, Harrison J, Abaloz E, Van Dyk S. Six year audit of cardiac arrests and medical emergency team calls in an outer metropolitan teaching hospital. BMJ. 2007;**335**(7631):1210-1212

[8] Buist M, DeVita M. How I nearly met my maker; A story of clinical futile cycles and survival. The Joint Commission Journal on Quality and Patient Safety. 2010;**36**(7):334-336

[9] Reason J. Managing the Risks of Organizational Accidents. Aldershot, Hampshire: Ashgate; 1997

[10] Palmieri PA, Delucia PR, Peterson LT, Ott TE, Green A. The anatomy and physiology of error in adverse health care events. Advances in Health Care Management. 2008;**7**: 33-68

[11] Australian Commission on Safety and Quality in Health Care. Literature Review: Medication Safety in Australia. Sydney: ACSQHC; 2013

[12] Australian Commission on Safety and Quality in Health Care. Safety and Quality Improvement Guide Standard 10: Preventing Falls and Harm from Falls (2012). Sydney. ACSQHC

[13] Haynes AB, Weiser TG, Berry WR, et al. A surgical safety checklist to reduce morbidity and mortality in a global population. The New England Journal of Medicine. 2009;**360**:491-499

[14] Wilson RM, Harrison BT, Gibberd RW, Hamilton JD. An analysis of the causes of adverse events from the Quality in Australian Health Care Study. The Medical Journal of Australia. 1999; **170**:411-415

[15] McQuillan P, Pilkington S, Allan A. Confidential enquiry into the quality of care before intensive care unit admission. BMJ. 1998;**316**:1853-1858

[16] Harrison GA, Hillman KM, Fulde GWO, Jacques TC. The need for undergraduate education in critical care. Anaesthesia and Intensive Care. 1999;**27**: 53-58

[17] Taylor D. Undergraduate procedural skills training in Victoria: Is it adequate? The Medical Journal of Australia. 1997; **171**:22-25

[18] Buist M, Jarmolovski E, Burton P, McGrath B, Waxman B, Meek R. Can interns manage clinical instability in hospital patients? A survey of recent graduates. Focus on Health Professional Education. 2001; **3**(3):20-28

[19] Cooper N. Medicine did not teach me what I really needed to know. BMJ. 2003;**327**(suppl):S190

[20] Mcdonald R. New initiative to improve undergraduate teaching in acute care. Student BMJ. 2004;**12**:68

[21] Stevens DP. Finding safety in medical education. Quality & Safety in Health Care. 2002;**11**:109-110

[22] Buist M. Predicting Hospital Crisis; Can we Do it? The Challenge of Predicting In-Hospital Iatrogenic Deaths in Medical Emergency Teams, Eds DeVita M, Hillman K. Bellomo R: Springer; 2011

[23] Stewart J. To call or not to call: A judgement of risk by pre-registration house officers. Medical Education. 2008; **42**:938-944

[24] Buist M, Burton P, Jarmolowski E, Bernard S, Waxman B. Recognising clinical instability in hospital patients before cardiac arrest or unplanned admission to intensive care: A pilot study. The Medical Journal of Australia. 1999;**171**:22-25

[25] Leape LL, Brennan TA, Laird N, Lawthers AG, Localio AR, Barnes BA, et al. The nature of adverse events in hospitalised patients: Results of the Harvard Medical Practice Study II. The New England Journal of Medicine. 1991; **324**:377-384

[26] Buist M, Bernard S, Anderson J. Epidemiology and prevention of unexpected in hospital deaths. The Surgeon: Journal of the Royal Colleges of Surgeons of Edinburgh and Ireland. 2003;**5**:265-268

[27] MERIT Study Investigators. Introduction of the medical emergency team (MET) system: A cluster randomised controlled study. Lancet. 2005;**365**:2091-2097

[28] Buist M. The rapid response team paradox: Why doesn't anyone call for help? Critical Care Medicine. 2008 Feb; **36**(2):634-636

[29] Marshall S, Shearer W, Buist M, Finnigan M, Kitto S, Hore T, et al. What stops hospital clinical staff from following protocols? An analysis of the incidence and factors behind the failure of bedside clinical staff to activate the Rapid Response System (RRS) in a multi-campus Australian metropolitan health care. BMJ Quality and Safety. 2012;**21**(7):569-575

[30] Kitto S, Marshall SD, McMillan SE, Shearer B, Buist M, Grant R, et al. Rapid response systems and collective (in) competence: An exploratory analysis of intraprofessional and interprofessional activation factors. Journal of Interprofessional Care. 2015;**29**(4): 340-346

[31] Buist M, Shearer W. Rapid response systems: A mandatory system of care or an optional extra for bedside clinical staff. Joint Commission Journal on Quality and Patient Safety. 2010;**36**(6): 263-265 241

[32] Jones DA, DeVita MA, Bellomo R. Rapid-response teams. The New England

Journal of Medicine. 2011;**365**(2): 139-146

[33] Maharaj R, Raffaele I, Wendon J. Rapid response systems: A systematic review and meta-analysis. Critical Care. 2015;**19**(1):1-15. DOI: 10.1186/s13054-015-0973-y

[34] Tirrkkonen J, Skrifvars MB, Tamminen T, Hillman K, Efendijev I, Aneman A, et al. Afferent limb failure revisited—A retrospective, international, multi centre, cohort study of delayed rapid response team calls. Resuscitation. 2020;**156**:6-14

[35] Flabouris A, Nandal S, Falbouris K, O'Connell A, Thompson C. Multi-tiered observation and response charts: Modifications and calls, to acutely deteriorating patients. PLoS One. 2015; **10**(12):e0145339

[36] Cuthbertson BH, Smith GB. A warning on early-warning scores. British Journal of Anaesthesia. 2007;**98**:704-706

[37] Edwards ED, Mason BW, Oliver A, Powell CV. Cohort study to test the predictability of the Melbourne criteria for the activation of the medical emergency team. Archives of Disease in Childhood. 2011;**96**:174-179

[38] Edwards ED, Powell CV, Mason BW, et al. Prospective cohort study to test the predictability of the Cardiff and Vale paediatric early warning system. Archives of Disease in Childhood. 2009;**94**:602-606

[39] Bodenheimer T, Sinsky C. From triple to quadruple aim: Care of the patient requires care of the provider. Annals of Family Medicine. 2014;**12**:573-576

[40] Barr DA. Science as superstition: Selecting medical students. Lancet. 2010; **376**:678-679

[41] Parker MH, Turner J, McGurgan P, et al. The difficult problem: Assessing medical students' professional attitudes and behaviour. The Medical Journal of Australia. 2010;**193**:662-664

[42] Bore M, Munro D, Powis D. A comprehensive model for the selection of medical students. Medical Teacher. 2009;**31**:1066-1072

[43] Wilson IG, Roberts C, Flynn EM, Griffin B. Only the best: Medical student selection in Australia. The Medical Journal of Australia. 2012;**196**(5):357

[44] Miller GE. The assessment of clinical skills/competence/performance. Academic Medicine. 1990;**65**(s9): S63-S67

[45] Harden RM, Stevenson M, Downie WW, Wison GM. Assessment of clinical competence using objective structured examinations. BMJ. 1975;**1**: 447-451

[46] Barman A. Critiques on the objective structured clinical examination. Annals of the Academy of Medicine, Singapore. 2005;**34**(8):478-482

[47] Garling P. Final report of the Special Commission of Inquiry: Acute Care Services in NSW Public Hospitals. Sydney: NSW Government; 2008. http://www.lawlink.nsw.gov.au/lawlink/Special_Projects/ll_splprojects.nsf/pages/acsi_finalreport

[48] Walker B. Final Report of the Special Commission of Inquiry into Campbelltown and Camden Hospitals. New South Wales Attorney General's Department: Sydney; 2004

[49] Hindle D, Braithwaite J, Travaglia J, Iedema R. Patient Safety: A Comparative Analysis of Eight Inquiries in Six Countries. Sydney: Centre for Clinical

Governance Research, University of New South Wales; 2006. http://www.cec.health.nsw.gov.au/pdf/PatientSafetyreportWEB3.pdf

[50] Report of the Mid Staffordshire NHS Foundation Trust Public Inquiry, Analysis of Evidence and Lessons Learned (Part 2). Vol. 2. London: The Stationery Office; 2013. www.midstaffspublicinquiry.com/report

[51] Learning from Bristol: The Report of the Public Inquiry into Children's Heart Surgery at the Bristol Royal Infirmary 1982–1995. London: Department of Health; 2001. ISBN: 0101520727. Available from the Stationery Office

[52] Davies G. Queensland Public Hospitals Commission of Inquiry. Brisbane: Queensland Public Hospitals Commission of Inquiry; 2005